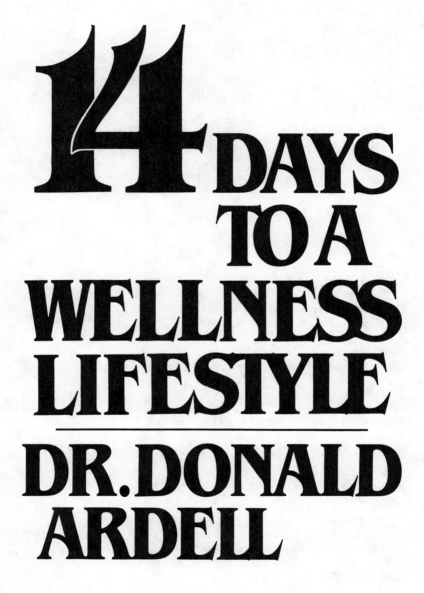

14 DAYS TO A WELLNESS LIFESTYLE

DR. DONALD ARDELL

© 1982 Donald B. Ardell

Published by Whatever Publishing, Inc.
158 E. Blithedale, Mill Valley, CA 94941

Cover design: Paul Hobson
Artwork: Nancy Olson

Manufactured in the United States of America

Library of Congress Cataloging in Publication Data
Ardell, Donald B.
    14 days to a wellness lifestyle.

    Bibliography: p. 299
    Includes index.
    1. Health.   2. Health behavior.   I. Title.
II. Title: Fourteen days to a wellness lifestyle.
RA776.A63   613   81-14824
ISBN 0-931432-11-1   AACR2

This book is dedicated to three friends who in different ways helped make wellness a viable option for many people:

Robert F. Allen of Morristown, New Jersey

William H. Hettler of Stevens Point, Wisconsin

John W. Travis of Mill Valley, California

Contents

Foreword

Don Ardell is one of the few people in the modern health care field who practices what he preaches. This book is a clear illustration of that fact. It makes it clear that we need to do more than talk about our wellness lifestyles — we need to live them. I have admired Don's work and life for a long, long time, and it is good to see it so well expressed in so relatively few pages.

In my own work, I have stressed the importance of building supportive environments for change. Don has been an important part of that supportive environment for many people, and this book should increase that support network a thousandfold. I hope many of you who are reading it will find ways to reach out and help others, for helping others can be one of the most important elements in creating and maintaining a positive wellness-oriented lifestyle.

It has been my experience that we, too often, try to do things all by ourselves and end up unsuccessful. My suggestion to the reader is that he/she become positively involved with other people in their wellness programs.

Through such positive involvement, there is a great deal that can be accomplished. In all of this, it is important that we recognize that our need for one another is not an obstacle to be overcome, but a virtue to be celebrated.

In the same way that Don Ardell's book can be helpful to us, so too can we be helpful to one another.

Robert F. Allen, Ph.D.
Human Resources Institute
Morristown, New Jersey

Introduction

> *How many times did it thunder before Franklin took the hint? How many apples fell on Newton's head before he took the hint? Nature is always hinting at us. It hints over and over again. And someday we take the hint.*
>
> —Robert Frost

Robert Frost was a wise man. Many of us have to experience a lot of thunder and apples crashing about us before we take Nature's hint. Like me, for instance.

Mark Twain also wrote something about thunder I think is absolutely terrific (I am not aware that Twain had anything to say about falling apples): "Thunder is good, thunder is impressive, but it is lightning that does the work."

My experience in promoting wellness has taught me that "hints" about health do not get the job done. People do not pay attention to thunder — it takes lightning to sell the kind of health approach that wellness has to offer.

Have you ever wondered why everybody in North America is not fit and healthy? Seriously. Why do you think weight control is a problem for more than half of all adults?

Why is junk food so popular? How come so many spend so much for tranquilizers and other drugs (including alcohol) to cope with the symptoms of stress? What explains the absence of exercise in the lives of over 100 million adults? How, in other words, do you account for the fact that very, very few people are at or anywhere close to the level of health that could be theirs?

Please circle your best guess.

A. Bad genes or other biological disadvantages.
B. Dreadful economic circumstances.
C. Awful health education in the homes and schools.
D. Society's infatuation with illness and disease.
E. Lack of interest in optimal health.

I think the *best* answer (all apply to some degree), the response that accounts for most cases of lost opportunity for genuine well-being, is "E," the lack of interest in optimal health.

Of course, the best *question* is: "Why is there such little interest?" Guess the answer to that one:

A. Information about health matters in general is dull.
B. Information on health topics usually focuses on illness, sickness, or disease.
C. Information regarding health issues dwells on the hazards and horrors of doing the "wrong things" (e.g., smoking).
D. People are encouraged in subtle and direct ways to view health as a medical matter.
E. The pursuit of "superhealth" entails too much sacrifice and insufficient fun.
F. The lifestyle required for advanced well-being requires too much effort, time, dedication, and sacrifice.
G. Most people assume that they are too old, too fat, too lazy, or a combination thereof to live in the manner required for wellness.

H. All of the above.

My guess would be "H."

This is a wellness book. Among other things, that means a special effort is made not to be dull about health, not to dwell upon disease, and not to focus on the awful wages of bad health habits. It also means that health will not be treated as a medical issue, and that you will be challenged to consider a wellness lifestyle as fun, practical, and within the reach of anyone. Nobody is too old, too fat, too lazy (or too ornery or too ugly) to enjoy the quest for wellness.

Do not look for ponderous scientific arguments, research evidence, or quoted medical advice. These can be useful on occasion, but for the most part that approach to health is a lot of thunder.

The approach here is to present 14 systematic steps to wellness that, like lightning, will help you get the job done. The "job," of course, is becoming all that you can be in terms of health — ambitiously defined. Unlike a lot of jobs, it is not hard work if approached properly. Indeed, a wellness lifestyle is more an avocation than a job. A wellness lifestyle is a pursuit chosen for the satisfactions it provides along the way as well as the product (advanced state of well-being) that comes from it.

In short, to get the job done, *you* need to provide the lightning. This book, therefore, has two purposes. The first purpose is to convey information. The second purpose is to help you to motivate yourself to choose and to maintain a wellness lifestyle — for a well lifetime.

The 14-Day plan you are about to begin is a progressive approach. The lessons of each Day are set up in order for you to gain maximum value from the concepts of succeeding Days. The Days gradually evolve in orientation from awareness to options to commitment to action.

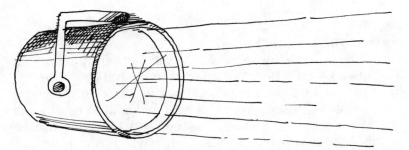

The book is definitely *not* about avoiding illness, getting better, or living longer. These will be positive side effects of pursuing wellness. The spotlight herein is on "super-health" — for its own sake, as its own reward.

The principles and opinions which account for the selection of the 14 Days are not advanced as comprehensive, exhaustive, ultimate truths supported by double-blind, crossover controls, absolutely scientific and 100 percent replicable by a ding-a-ling investigator, myself included. In the wonderful world of lifestyle change, not all the variables can be controlled or explained. My experience strongly suggests that the system works — which is the ultimate test.

Reading *14 Days* should not take more than twenty minutes daily, and more likely fifteen. This is a deliberate program feature — please do not do more than one lesson per day. If you are stuck someplace and this is the only reading material available, then skip to Part Two (Wellness Innovations), or Part Three (Wellness Honor Roll). This allows you sufficient time to ponder aspects of each day, to maintain brevity so you do not get mired in boring detail, and to leave plenty of time (i.e., 23 hrs. and 45 min.) to *practice* other aspects of healthy living on your own.

As each day progresses, you might find three things happening: (1) your information or awareness level is rising; (2) your motivation to pursue whole-person excellence is increasing; and (3) your capacity to sustain a wellness lifestyle beyond the initial 14 Days is being strengthened.

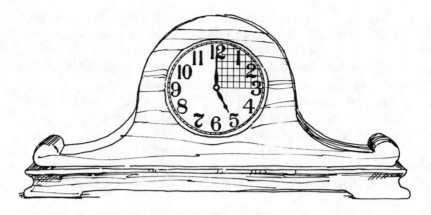

Each chapter begins with a statement of purpose that expresses the goal of that particular Day. There is a checklist at the back of the book — you are asked to mark the completion of each lesson as you go along. I have sprinkled the book with similar little tasks and exercises to increase your participation in the processes of shaping a wellness lifestyle. These activities will increase your enjoyment of and dedication to completion of the 14 Days.

Not every Day is equally important. I admit it — and besides, how's an author to measure the relative use of each lesson? — weigh the chapters? hire a jury? ask his friends? The first method isn't scientific. The second is expensive and questionable: would a San Francisco consensus hold water in Des Moines? And, the third approach is impossible — my friends can't read.

However, if you insist on a rank order of important days — the most important is Day One, followed by Days Two through 14! But remember, that's because I was already into wellness when I wrote this book. So, want to know what I really think? I think everybody will have her/his own favorite Days, and that there will be great variation in the choices different folks make — depending on what issues are encountered in the real world as they reach each Day's discussion.

So, don't skip any Days. If, when you finish, you want to extend the program a bit, feel free to write your own extra Day or two to wellness. Do me a favor and send me a copy, in care of the publisher. It just may be exactly what I need to stop chain-smoking (I'm kidding).

I hope you enjoy this approach immensely, and that it is of use as you pursue your unique quest and pathways to whole-person excellence.

Remember — don't settle for thunder.

FURTHER HINTS FOR THE 14-DAY PLAN

I have incorporated a few unusual techniques in the layout of this book. You may find them rather odd. Either way, here is an explanation of what to expect and the method behind the madness.

I think you will derive more from this and any other book that treats the sensitive and personal subject of life-style attitudes and behaviors if you participate and enjoy the process. So, I threw in a few out-of-the-ordinary things to keep you alert.

One is the time factor already mentioned. Fifteen minutes should be sufficient for most of the 14 Days. Of course, some Days you might have to read real fast. However, on other occasions you can move your lips as you go along and finish with time to spare.

Another technique concerns the stated purpose of the Day's program. If, after finishing a lesson, you do not think the point(s) was persuasively made, then you can: (1) read it again, or (2) consider me a turkey! I put extra effort into producing a persuasive text — no writer wants to be called a turkey.

Another technique that is a part of this opus is a two-week calendar printed at the back of this book. When you finish a Day, you check that accomplishment right in the book. As time goes by and you make your way through, you see at a glance a record of your movement and growing awareness. Just entering the check should in itself be a satisfying and reinforcing little experience. You will be reminded to make your inimitable mark at the end of each Day's reading.

There are sometimes quotes at the beginning, jokes at the end and, occasionally, drawings in between. Who said that health enhancement had to hurt or bore you? But my favorite device for keeping you involved and insuring that you profit from this close encounter with wellness is the music to accompany each Day's reading. Music? Am I being serious? Absolutely. Now, of course, I cannot stroll from the page to sing "Happy Wellness to You" or something like that, but I can recommend that you play certain masterpieces as you go along. You do not have to do this to experience the 14-Day Plan, but there are four reasons why I believe you ought to try it. Maybe five.

Without going into a long story on the research evidence and the history of the work being done in the field of "superlearning," just be aware that there are four basic claims for the method.* Here they are: (1) music activates the right hemisphere of the brain for greater creativity, intuition, and imagination; (2) it increases one's ability to synthesize and recall material; (3) it deepens the capacity to relax and focus on the issues being introduced; and (4) it promotes enthusiasm for the material presented. Since there is lots of evidence that humans use only about ten percent of their brain capacity, you almost have to pay attention to this stuff. I mean, if the method (or, more accurately, my variation on it) gets you no further than twenty percent of your potential, that's a 100 percent advance! You will have doubled your effectiveness. Anyway, I mentioned a fifth reason to try the music idea. The fifth reason is that even if the other claims do not work out, you will get to enjoy the magnificent beauty of some of the loveliest sounds of the past few centuries.

---

*Sheila Ostrander and Lynn Schroeder, *Superlearning* (Delta: New York, 1979).

All musical selections are personal favorites of mine. A few meet the criteria for "superlearning" purposes (i.e., a largo or largetto beat of 40-60 and 60-66 beats per minute, respectively). However, this was not my major consideration. The prime factor was my love for and desire to share the music I enjoy so much.

The selection recommended for each Day is listed on the last page of this book (page 378). So, get out the classical records and tapes — and charm yourself. If the suggested selection is not conveniently available, use another Day's choice, or one of your own that creates a special mood of fulfillment and serenity.

Part One is the heart of the book — and the section to which the title refers. The larger eleven-point type signifies as much. If you were to read only this portion, you would derive full value from your investment of time and money in the book. Part Two is a bonus, of sorts. It evidences the nature of and variations in the wellness movement. It, too, could stand alone. It is in ten-point print to suggest that it supports but does not distract from the *14 Days* to be mastered. The last section of the book is Part Three, the Honor Roll of Recommended Readings. Consider this a special bonus, not vital to your near-term program but useful later on. To keep the *14 Days* program from appearing at first glance as encyclopedic in size or voluminous in discourse, Part Three was set in nine-point type! So, get out your magnifying glass. Enjoy.

Part One

14 Days to a
Wellness Lifestyle

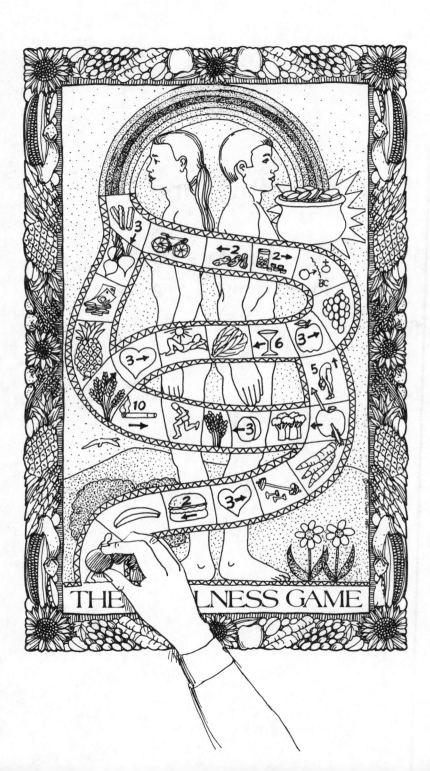

THE WELLNESS GAME

Day One

Learn The Rules Of
The Wellness Game *

Purpose: At the end of this day you will know what wellness is about. That's it! Nothing complicated — just a few basics about what health *really* is to steer you toward "bigger things" in the days to come.

Think of wellness as a game. A "game" is defined as "an activity engaged in for diversion or amusement." It is also "a procedure or strategy for gaining an end." It is "synonymous with fun" (Webster).

Why should wellness, a lifestyle for pursuing your optimal potentials, be other than enjoyable — or fun? A game? No reason.

Consider the elements of a game for just a moment. Games have rules, penalties/rewards, onlookers, players, goals, agreements, winners/losers, expectations, adversaries, uncertainties, and skill requirements. Some people have innate advantages for playing the game; some have to

*The idea of wellness as a game with rules, expectations, and so on reflects to some extent the work of Klaus Hilgers of Morristown, New Jersey, the Director of the Well Being Workshops. I want to acknowledge Klaus for his creative adaptation of organizational effectiveness and group-process techniques to communications about wellness lifestyles.

practice more than others to reach the same level.

Wellness has all these characteristics. Only the forms are different from the other games you know and play.

To play the Wellness Game, you have to choose or agree to participate — which leads to the first rule of the Wellness Game: *Make a commitment. Decide to play.* Agree that this is what you want to do. Begin.

In a way, you are very close to such a start. After all, you bought, borrowed, or stole this book. So why not begin the 14 Days by putting in writing your decision to play the Wellness Game.

In the space provided, write: "I am committed to playing the Wellness Game." Sign your name to this agreement.

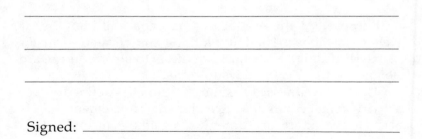

Signed: _____

You just made wellness real. Games, though associated with play, need not be frivolous to be workable, valuable, and fun.

The rest of the Day's reading provides a few more details about rules — or suggestions — for enjoying and winning the Wellness Game.

Here is the bottom line for the game: Wellness is a lifestyle approach for realizing your best possibilities for well-being. The key is lifestyle — the range of actions under your control, such as how you eat, exercise, manage stress, think of the medical system and, in general, treat your body and perceive the world around you. Environment is important, heredity plays a key role, and the health care system has an impact, but only lifestyle is under your direct influence. For this reason, the emphasis in the Wellness Game is on all the elements that fit in the lifestyle category that affect well-being. Well-being, in this sense, encompasses all aspects of your existence — physical, emotional, mental, and spiritual.

The name given to this game, *wellness,* was first used a decade ago by the late Halbert L. Dunn, a physician. I never met him, but I learned about him by reading his books and articles and visiting places where he lived and worked. Dr. Dunn was an important influence for me and for the wellness movement which he helped create.

I like the word "wellness," because it serves as a substitute for another word that everybody knows but usually misuses, "health!"

Most people think of health as a state you are in when you are not sick, without disease, free of pain. In other words, health is associated with the absence of something — illness.

This perspective is *hazardous* to your health and makes The Game more difficult. When you believe this, the best you can hope for is not to be sick. As a result, you may limit yourself to achieving the minimal requirements for non-illness.

The alternative, which wellness invites, is to describe health as having a positive dimension. This encompasses *levels* of well-being, or stages and positions along a continuum of whole-person functioning, that encourage pictures of optimal existence. Note the difference in the two perspectives. In the first case, health as non-illness, the best position available is "not sick."

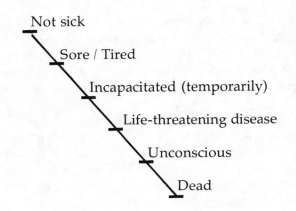

Not sick

Sore / Tired

Incapacitated (temporarily)

Life-threatening disease

Unconscious

Dead

There are, of course, thousands of ways to describe the multiple states of illness that can occur between dead and not sick. But under the prevailing model, there is a near absence of awareness, interest, discussion, and insight into the states of health above the line of not sick. In my view, this has serious if subtle consequences.

I will give you a personal example. A few months ago, I went to a physician for a standard physical examination. I was not ill or concerned about any difficulties that a diagnosis would reveal. I simply needed the usual test in order to have my private pilot's license renewed. At the time, by the way, I was in great shape. I had trained over a year for the San Francisco Marathon. My heart rate was low, weight was down, and so forth. I was pretty pleased with the way things stood. In fact, I expected a compliment from the doctor — you know, some crack like, "You are in great shape for an eighty-year-old guy." Instead, the doctor looked at the test results, then at me, and said: "Well, I could not find anything wrong. I would say that you are medically uninteresting." I thanked him, paid the bill, and left. I wondered about his comment on the way home. Is "medically uninteresting" what lies beyond the state of "not sick?"

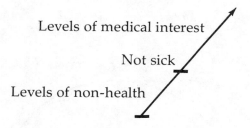

Levels of medical interest

Not sick

Levels of non-health

Of course not. Unfortunately, doctors have not been trained in medical school to promote health. As a result, they fail to recognize it when they see it. The idea of wellness is to help *you* recognize, pursue, and achieve a state of health beyond "not sick" and "medically uninteresting." There truly is a great deal more to health than the absence of illness or the presence of medical noninterest. There are terms, phrases, images, and other classifications which can be placed on the continuum. In the Days to come, I will suggest a few possibilities and encourage you to develop your own expressions or words for these positive states.

For today, what you need to acknowledge is that the term "health" is not often used in the best and fullest sense of the word, and that wellness is a term that embodies new parameters and expectations of well-being. Here are a few of them.

· A wellness lifestyle has five dimensions: self-responsibility, nutritional awareness, physical fitness, stress management, and environmental sensitivity. All five areas are equally important. However, self-responsibility is "more equal" (thanks, George Orwell). Without an awareness of and full commitment to the reality that you are the prime cause for what goes well or poorly regarding your life in general and health in particular, you are not likely to want to invest the time and energy required to pursue knowledge and practice in the other four dimensions. The following diagram depicts the five dimensions of wellness, and notes the central role of self-responsibility.

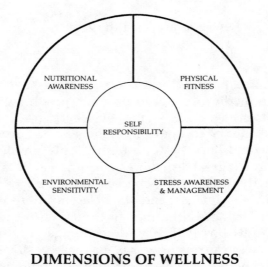

DIMENSIONS OF WELLNESS

· Wellness is a positive approach. The reasons for pursuing wellness are always related to satisfactions, payoffs, pleasures, and the like — not sickness avoidance or life extension. The latter are likely side effects, but not sufficient in themselves to motivate and sustain health-enhancing habit patterns. So, do not look for information in this book about all the frightful things that will happen to you if you do not practice wellness — such as: blindness, eyes crossing, a peevish and morose disposition, bed-wetting, unnatural appetites, hair growth on the palms, and other symptoms of self-abuse. Such negative appeals seldom work — people will always think of some way to outwit negative admonitions. You have heard of the youngster who, when caught fondling himself, was warned that such behavior will cause blindness — to which his response was: "Can I do it until I need glasses?" In wellness, the emphasis is on near-term pleasures from choosing the right path, not on long-term penalties for wrong-doing.

· Wellness lifestyles must be unique to each person. No guru or expert can tell you what to do or how to do it. Your style, opportunities, situation, and resources are unlike those of anyone else. Enjoy the quest for your own unique pathways to excellence.

Wellness includes physical health *and* emotional/mental well-being, which leads to an overall sense of satisfaction with your reasons for being. The physical aspect is probably the least important aspect of wellness, but it is a pathway toward the greater psychological and spiritual returns.

Four different terms can be used to describe popular lifestyle choices in a progression from "superhealth" or high-level wellness to minimal functioning or low-level worseness. In between these two extremes are middle-level mediocrity or "muddling through" (the most common lifestyle pattern), and a lifestyle approach of isolated acts toward becoming healthier. This last behavior syndrome is called "intermediate-level omnibus tinkering with health." Naturally, all of us act at times in ways that are characteristic of each lifestyle pattern. Yet, we all favor one of the four.

Where would you place yourself on the continuum? Which of the following is most reflective of your current lifestyle pattern?

WORSENESS/WELLNESS LIFESTYLE CONTINUUM

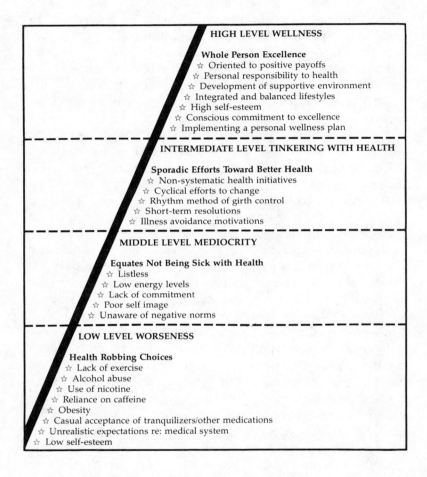

HIGH LEVEL WELLNESS

Whole Person Excellence
☆ Oriented to positive payoffs
☆ Personal responsibility to health
☆ Development of supportive environment
☆ Integrated and balanced lifestyles
☆ High self-esteem
☆ Conscious commitment to excellence
☆ Implementing a personal wellness plan

INTERMEDIATE LEVEL TINKERING WITH HEALTH

Sporadic Efforts Toward Better Health
☆ Non-systematic health initiatives
☆ Cyclical efforts to change
☆ Rhythm method of girth control
☆ Short-term resolutions
☆ Illness avoidance motivations

MIDDLE LEVEL MEDIOCRITY

Equates Not Being Sick with Health
☆ Listless
☆ Low energy levels
☆ Lack of commitment
☆ Poor self image
☆ Unaware of negative norms

LOW LEVEL WORSENESS

Health Robbing Choices
☆ Lack of exercise
☆ Alcohol abuse
☆ Use of nicotine
☆ Reliance on caffeine
☆ Obesity
☆ Casual acceptance of tranquilizers/other medications
☆ Unrealistic expectations re: medical system
☆ Low self-esteem

In Day Two, you will have an opportunity to decide which of these four patterns best describes your current lifestyle. The test is only of historic interest. What really matters is where you decide to go in the time ahead.

14 Days will help you choose and sustain your own program leading you to the top of this lifestyle continuum. You will never regret it.

· You can practice wellness at any point in the life cycle. It applies as much to the old as the young, to the poor as to the affluent, to the sick and dying as to the well. Wellness is more an attitude or a context in which to perceive your life and purposes than it is a position to be in.

· Wellness is not the same as holistic health, prevention, or medical self-care. There are similarities and consistencies, and wellness efforts can fit with any or all of the above. But the thrust is different in each case. Holistic health is usually oriented to treatment, prevention to illness avoidance, and medical self-care to layperson capacity to identify and attend to minor health problems. Wellness, as mentioned, is targeted to the enjoyable, lifelong quest for attainable peaks of optimal whole-person functioning as its own reward.

Living a wellness lifestyle is never an accident: it is a consequence of making a deliberate choice to live at the heights. To get there, however, you must realize that there are larger forces which must be considered and managed.

One of these forces is the larger culture(s) of which you are a part. Day Four is devoted to helping you identify, analyze, and prepare to deal with those parts of your environment which have immense consequence to your prospects for wellness living. Personal determination is not enough. Group support is also needed — at home, work and elsewhere.

There are just a few other "rules" (or suggestions) that make the Wellness Game more fun and increase the chances that you will win big at it. One is to know what it means in a physical sense to be at the top of the Wellness Continuum (you will read about this in Day Four); another is to have a clear picture or set of images regarding what psychological or spiritual wellness is all about (see Day Five).

By the end of 14 Days, you will have a complete account of what I think are the rules (or principles, guides, keys, etc.) and techniques for playing the Wellness Game. You will also possess something more important — the ability and interest to create your own rules to guide you for the next 14 Days, and weeks, months, years, and decades after that. That capacity, that talent, that orientation, will be invaluable. Treasure and cultivate it.

This is it for Day One. You are now aware that there is more to health than non-sickness or illness. You already have a good sense for the general direction of a wellness outlook, and a measure of confidence that you can act accordingly.

When you think of wellness as a game, the pursuit of advanced well-being becomes a lifelong no-lose contest in which you get to win every day, find continuing meaning, and experience recurring satisfaction. A wellness lifestyle will always encourage you to think of yourself as a whole, complete, and sufficient being. Thanks for "sharing" this first day. (Some people believe that we Californians share too much. I have friends in the Midwest who think that it takes six Californians to screw in a light bulb. Really! One to turn the bulb and five to "share" in the experience. This is not true. Four of us can handle it nicely.)

Please check off Day One on the calendar at the back of the book.

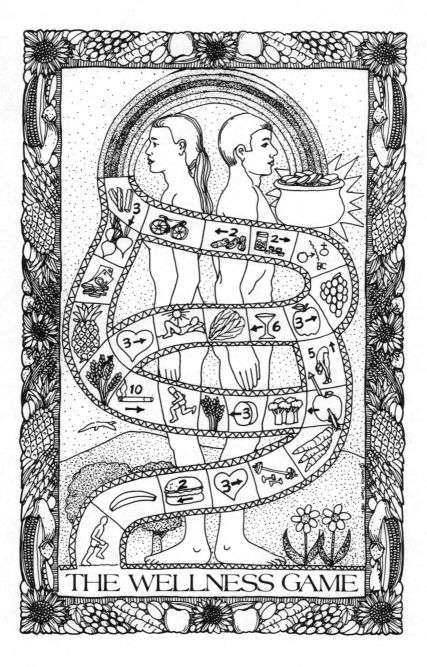

THE WELLNESS GAME

Day Two

Test Yourself For Temporary Placement On The Worseness/Wellness Continuum

Purpose: At the end of this day you will have a bench mark or measure of where you are at the start of your wellness program.

In the discussion during Day One, I described the wellness lifestyle, contrasting it with the limited picture that most people have of health (i.e., "not sick"). Today should be a special treat for you. You get to take a test, and any score you get is OK. Really! You see, it actually does not matter a whole lot where you are now; what truly counts is where you want to be in the future. This test will help you decide. It will also give you some measures that you can use later to chart your progress. With these bench marks, you will notice how well you are doing in the near term, which will add considerably to your satisfaction in moving ahead to new levels.

When you finish the test, I will interpret the results. You will learn more about the four patterns of lifestyles sketched in Day One, and see where you are — for the moment — on the Worseness/Wellness Continuum.

Enjoy the test — if in doubt, give yourself the benefit of

any hesitation or uncertainty. The answers, to tell you the inside scoop, matter less than the consciousness raising that the questions are designed to evoke.

THE WORSENESS/WELLNESS CONTINUUM TEST

SELF-RESPONSIBILITY

1. My health is affected more by what I do or do not do than it is by doctors, circumstances, fate, the gods, drugs, hospitals, and other factors outside of my control.

☐ *Yes, I agree*   ☐ *No, I disagree*   ☐ *Not sure*

2. A number of interesting and worthwhile wellness, holistic-health, prevention, and medical self-help books have been published in recent years. Have you read any?

☐ *Yes*   ☐ *No*

3. If the pay was attractive and other considerations were favorable, but the job being offered posed a threat to your health (i.e., would bring you into contact with potentially carcinogenic chemicals, toxic people, or hazardous pollutants such as arsenic, asbestos, benzine, coal-combustion products, nickel compounds, dioxin, chloroform, trichloroethylene, carbon tetrachloride, radiation, synthetic estrogens, vinyl chloride, silica, iron, benzene, beryllium, dusts, fumes, mists, gases, and cigarette smoke, cigar and pipe smokers), would you turn the job down?

☐ *Yes*   ☐ *No*   ☐ *Not sure*

4. Drug companies spend billions for TV and other ads pushing pills for all manner of aches, pains, and disorders (real as well as fabricated) known to men, women, beasts, and combinations thereof. All are designed to mask or alleviate symptoms and other signals of bodily distress. Are you aware that these "remedies" often aggravate the illness condition — and do absolutely nothing to help you understand and deal with the underlying source of the problem?

☐ *Yes*   ☐ *No*

5. Can you embrace and live the philosophy that the quality of your life, as well as your satisfaction and fulfillment in life, is not forever dependent upon your circumstances (e.g., the parents or mate you are/were stuck with, your job or school, your physical and economic assets or deprivations and the like)?

☐ *Yes*   ☐ *No*

6. Do you keep any kind of a written journal, diary, plan, logbook, etc., for purposes of inventorying your resources, setting goals, tracking your moods, charting your progress, and generally staying in touch with your own evolution?

☐ *Yes*   ☐ *No*

7. Have you made a conscious commitment to your own well-being? (It's easy to slide into poor condition and awful habits as you get older — no special awareness of doing so is required; experiencing wellness and getting "superhealthy" by taking responsibility for your life and shaping a life-enriching behavior and attitude pattern in each wellness dimension requires a conscious commitment to your best potentials.)

☐ *Yes*   ☐ *No*

8. Do you make an effort to avoid waiting around for, or looking ahead to, "happy times" — Christmas, holidays, Friday afternoons, moments of athletic heroism, lovemaking, etc. — to the extent that what you do most of the time seems routine and dull? (One objective of a wellness lifestyle is to expand your power to enjoy more of all life experiences.)

☐ *Yes*   ☐ *No*

9. Are you aware of the massive overuse and misuse that is reflected in the expensive, high-technology, hospital-centered, doctor-dominated, and illness-focused health or medical care system? Do you have a general sense for what modern medicine can and cannot do for various kinds of health problems? When you do have encounters with doctors and nurses, do you ask lots of questions and

reserve for yourself final decision-making authority as to whether a recommended medication or treatment is really necessary?

☐ *Yes*   ☐ *No*

10. Do you recognize that difficult, even "crisis," moments and events in your life can be (and probably have been) special opportunities for new growth and valuable change?

☐ *Yes*   ☐ *No*

Please score two points for each "yes" response to these first ten questions.

NUTRITIONAL AWARENESS

11. Do or did your parents, friends, or others use sweets or other foods as a reward? — e.g., "Clean your plate, dearie, and I'll take you out for a chocolate slurpee."

☐ *Yes*   ☐ *No*

12. Do you use food as entertainment, with a greater concern for pleasing your senses than nourishing your cells?

☐ *Yes*   ☐ *No*

13. Do you regularly consume such foods as processed meats (high in nitrites, fat, salt, and monosodium glutamate, among other digestive ghastlies), colas, sugar-loaded cereals and desserts, white bread, and fast foods?

☐ *Yes*   ☐ *No*

14. Do you combine high-energy conversation (e.g., arguing, debating, or other emotional expressions) with eating?

☐ *Yes*   ☐ *No*

15. Studies in recent years have strongly indicated what exercise physiologists have been saying for some time: that exercise usually *depresses* appetite; that dieting without exercise causes harmful loss of *lean* tissue; and that standard life-insurance-company tables for assessing "ideal" body weight create more harm than good (by suggesting

that it is normal to get fatter with increasing age). Are these findings surprising to you in that you did not know this already?

☐ *Yes*   ☐ *No*

16. Considering the importance of nutrition to health ("bad" food patterns are a major factor in at least six of the ten major chronic diseases; "good" food patterns are an essential element in achieving physical excellence), is it reasonable or acceptable that corporations, schools, and hospitals do *not* offer regular diet-pattern profiles for interested workers, patients, and students? (In having such an analysis, you would be asked to record everything you ate for one week and from this you would receive a written report showing your caloric intake, vitamin/mineral levels, roughage consumption, percentage of fat/protein/complex versus simple carbohydrate usage, and recommendations for adjustments, if appropriate.)

☐ *Yes*   ☐ *No*

17. Many of us have a tendency to eat when we are bored, depressed, upset, or otherwise out of sorts with ourselves. Is this a problem for you, and a major source of poor food habits?

☐ *Yes*   ☐ *No*

18. The rationale for food additives is to counter spoilage. Are you satisfied with the necessity of, as well as government safeguards for, varied chemical additives?

☐ *Yes*   ☐ *No*

19. Is your idea of a natural-foods gourmet treat a six-pack and a "Big Mac"?

☐ *Yes*   ☐ *No*

20. Would you agree with a statement to the effect that food preferences (that is, your likes and dislikes) are innate and cannot be learned or relearned?

☐ *Yes*   ☐ *No*

Please add two points to your score for each "no" response which you checked in this section.

PHYSICAL FITNESS

21. Are you aware of your own resting pulse, your target training heart rate for optimal aerobic conditioning, your heart recovery rate, your vital capacity, and your percent of body fat relative to lean muscle tissue?

☐ *Yes (all of the above)* ☐ *No (none or just a few)*

22. Do you participate in more sporting events than you observe?

☐ *Yes* ☐ *No*

23. Consider the reading you enjoy regularly in the sports category. Is most of this reading participant-oriented (e.g., *The Runner, Bike World*) rather than spectator-oriented material (e.g., *Sports Illustrated*)?

☐ *Yes* ☐ *No*

24. Are you familiar with minimal standards of adequacy for exercise, and do you exceed these measures in your regular activity routines?

☐ *Yes* ☐ *No*

25. Do you have a general appreciation for the benefits of different kinds of exercise, such as endurance, strength, and flexibility, and do you have a balance of such activity in your exercise routine?

☐ *Yes* ☐ *No*

26. Do you supplement your aerobic workouts with warm-up and warm-down periods?

☐ *Yes* ☐ *No*

27. Do you enjoy whatever it is you do for regular physical conditioning?

☐ *Yes* ☐ *No*

28. Do you feel really good about the way your body looks?

☐ *Yes* ☐ *No*

29. Do you belong to a "Y", health club, athletic program, and/or a group of one kind or another that supports and motivates you in getting regular exercise?

☐ *Yes* ☐ *No*

30. Do you derive satisfaction from going out of your way to experience "extra" exercise beyond your normal routines? For example, do you climb stairs rather than ride escalators, other things being the same (i.e., when you are not carrying a heavy suitcase, in a hurry, or in the company of a sedentary person who needs your arm to lean on)?
☐ *Yes*   ☐ *No*

Credit yourself with two points for each "yes" response to the last ten questions.

STRESS AWARENESS AND MANAGEMENT

31. Are you aware that you have the potential to moderate your blood pressure, blood flow, heart rate, glandular secretions, muscular tensions, and the temperatures in your hands and feet?
☐ *Yes*   ☐ *No*

32. Can you recall an instance in the past week when you used deep breathing or progressive muscle control?
☐ *Yes*   ☐ *No*

33. Are you familiar with more than one technique for managing stress? Do you regularly employ a method of centering or balancing yourself in times of perceived stressful circumstances?
☐ *Yes*   ☐ *No*

34. Are you clear that you create your own feelings, that your continued reaction to a stressful event is a matter of your choice, and that you have the power — if you are willing and able to employ it — to choose how you will feel about *any* event?
☐ *Yes*   ☐ *No*

35. Are you alert to stress symptoms, such as trying to do more than one thing at a time (e.g., brushing your teeth on the pot, reading and eating), fingernail chewing, cold hands and feet, toe tapping, muscle twitches, tension, or

aches (especially in the neck and shoulders), clammy hands, and perspiring while at rest?

☐ Yes   ☐ No

36. Do you recover quickly from the effects of emotion-charged events (e.g., witnessing an accident, hearing terrible news, etc.)? Put another way, are you a stabilizing influence when others around you might be close to panic?

☐ Yes   ☐ No

37. Do you sleep well?

☐ Yes   ☐ No

38. Do you use imagery, visualizations, affirmations, or other advanced techniques to achieve desired states, such as serenity or a higher level of consciousness for creativity?

☐ Yes   ☐ No

39. Do you find it easy to express a full range of emotions (joy, sorrow, anger, laughter)?

☐ Yes   ☐ No

40. Can you experience failure without great upset? Can you usually perceive in any setback the seeds of new opportunities, as invitations for new growth and directions?

☐ Yes   ☐ No

Again, please credit yourself with two points for each "yes" response.

ENVIRONMENTAL SENSITIVITY

41. Do you realize that the predominant messages of the culture, the slant of the media, and the signals of societal norms often make low-level worseness habits seem normal (e.g., ashtrays on tables in restaurants) and even attractive? Can you sense that a vast number of subtle reinforcements for destructive behaviors, over a long period of time, can exert a powerful, inhibitory effect on your prospects for wellness?

☐ Yes   ☐ No

42. Do you regularly enjoy hearty belly laughs? Can you recall recent instances when you had a laugh on you? Is your sense of humor above average, in your opinion?

Check "yes" to this question if all three are affirmative. Laughter is a key to emotional health. It also has a healing power. Laughter relaxes muscles, relieves pains, fights off infections, reduces inflammations, and makes you feel good all over. An excellent source of mirth is yourself — it helps a lot not to take yourself too seriously. If you laugh hard and often enough, you will surely kill off anything unpleasant that might be growing inside of you.

☐ *Yes*　　☐ *No*

43. Do you have a reasonably clear picture of what optimal health can look like for you? Besides not being sick, can you imagine how your potentials for well-being might make you feel, look, act, respond in relation to others — and to your "old self"?

☐ *Yes*　　☐ *No*

44. Do you truly enjoy the activities in which you now spend most of your time? Answer "yes" if you would be doing these or similar activities if you had plentiful alternatives — or if you knew you were going to be dead in three days.

☐ *Yes*　　☐ *No*

45. Do you have a positive self-concept that *you*, over time, have developed for yourself? Is this identity basically untainted by negative images shaped by parents, friends, teachers, or others?

☐ *Yes*　　☐ *No*

46. Do you make an effort to acknowledge your own uniqueness, resisting the "comparison trap" of wishing you looked like, were as young as, achieved as much as, or were the equal of someone else?

☐ *Yes*　　☐ *No*

47. Are you generally willing to function assertively in order to realize your needs? Do you operate from strength, rejecting victim tendencies in the way you deal with co-

workers and friends? (Examples would be an ability not to "go along" if you don't want to, not to say "yes" if you desire "no," not to continue a communication or relationship if not interested, and not to eat something to please Granny or anyone else.)

☐ *Yes*   ☐ *No*

48. Do you live and work in supportive environments? Are most of your friends interested in healthy lifestyles? Supportive environments are characterized as surroundings, organizations, and networks providing (among other things) open communications, the keeping of agreements, valued contributions, respect for excellence, a sense of family, and the plentiful expression of love and joy.

☐ *Yes*   ☐ *No*

49. Do you make an effort to moderate your possessions and your impact upon natural resources?

☐ *Yes*   ☐ *No*

50. Do you make a point to eliminate self-destructive concepts such as blame, worry, guilt, jealousy, and boredom?

☐ *Yes*   ☐ *No*

That's it — the test is over. Please add two points again for each of the "yes" responses to the questions in the environmental-sensitivity section. Total your score.

There are four categories in which you can place yourself. None of them is totally accurate, unfortunately, but each is fun, so what the hell.

If your overall score is between eighty and one hundred, you ought to write a book. Seriously, you are doing super well. The 14-Day program will be a real pleasure for you. You will be reading about and practicing approaches that are totally consistent with your current lifestyle — keep up the impressive performance. I am pleased for you.

Perhaps your score was between sixty-four and seventy-eight. (Note the precision in these figures — note this, but do not take it too seriously.) This qualifies for another lifestyle classification reserved for those who come close to wellness, but fall short. If you are in this category, you probably go back and forth on the wellness continuum from not sick to kind-of-well to a-little-not-well, and so forth — never advancing very far beyond the neutral point. If you diet, you probably go up and down on the scales, gaining and then losing weight, practicing what might be called the rhythm method of girth control. The name of this lifestyle? — "Intermediate-Level Omnibus Tinkering with Health."

Maybe your score was between fifty and sixty-two. If so, your lifestyle is not so bad, but it is not exactly terrific for wellness purposes. This range indicates you sort of muddle through, not doing anything really bizarre and self-destructive but not staying up nights reading about optimal health, either. This lifestyle is, in my opinion, the single most popular pattern in the U.S. and Canada. I call it "Middle-Level Mediocrity."

OK, so maybe your score was below fifty. Does this mean you are on the Interstate-to-Ruin, the fast track to an early demise? Probably. But you need not get stuck there. Some of my wellness-oriented friends who are at the top of the continuum today once were experts at this lifestyle pattern, which I call "Low-Level Worseness." Not to worry. It is not true that the only cure for you is embalming fluid. Take another look at the continuum chart introduced on the first day. The best reason for moving up is that there is more satisfaction in being in the wellness phase.

The test has three purposes: (1) to have you look at your lifestyle practices in relation to four generalized patterns, which should encourage you to assess what pattern you want to pursue (naturally, the wellness option!); (2) to give you a bench mark sense of where you are at the moment, which makes it easier to notice progress as the days go by; and (3) to arouse your curiosity about issues in the five wellness dimensions.

Thanks for being a good sport in taking the test. Pondering your position on each question is more consequential than how you did on the test. You are ahead of where you were two days ago.

Here is a story with a non-wellness moral about a boy with no body! Though a happy fellow, very popular, smart, and totally committed to a healthy lifestyle, the lack of a body was a considerable handicap. All he had, since birth, was a head. Despite this difficulty, which would have dispirited most, he experienced a surprisingly full youth. A member of the debate club, the choir, and vice-president of his class, he was your average, all-American boy, except that he lacked a body (which people hardly noticed once they got to know him).

Then, one day, it happened. A girlfriend, with whom he was particularly enamored, mentioned that she really liked him, admired his achievements, and was greatly impressed with his wellness lifestyle, etc., but she wished he had a body. Though he was not upset at the time, the seeds of dissatisfaction had been planted. He was no longer content with his head. Now he wanted a body. Furthermore, he decided to take action to get one.

To do so, he used a multitude of holistic techniques. Oh yes, doctors said it could not be done, that it was medically impossible, but he was not dissuaded. He read all the books on growing a body (there were not many), relentlessly employed will power, hypnosis, affirmations, imagery, and tried dozens of "New Age" modalities. Within three months, it was evident that he was indeed growing a body. The medical community was astonished. The news services picked up the story; the boy was invited to appear on "The Johnny Carson Show," "Sixty Minutes," and "That's Incredible." He ignored them all, maintained his privacy, and continued his quest for a body. In another three months of channeled energy flows, psychic empowerments, and good vibrations, his body was complete. It was beautiful — lean and shaped for high performance. On the first day with his new body, he went out jogging. He wanted to impress the young lady whose idle remark about no body started all this in the first place. But, a tragic thing happened. He was run over by a U-Haul truck.

Know the moral of this tale? Quit while you're a head.

Actually, you should not quit when you are ahead (or behind). There is no future in it. As Parkinson suggested, "The future lies ahead."

You are already ahead because you have a body. Even if your body has been stuck in low-level worseness, middle-level mediocrity, or intermediate-level omnibus tinkering, that period is over. In the next 14 Days, you will advance to the wellness end of the continuum. You do not have to grow a new body. Just reshape the old one.

Please, with a flourish, mark Day Two as complete. See you tomorrow.

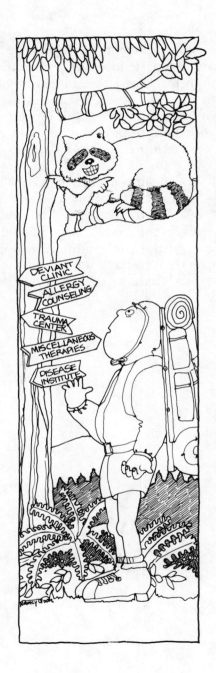

Day Three

Develop A Realistic Perspective On The Medical System

Purpose: To develop a perspective on the medical system that will complement your evolving wellness lifestyle. You should develop a sense for the problems which characterize the medical system, what actual capabilities doctors, hospitals, drugs, and the rest have to offer in treating illness, and what role the medical system plays in positive health.

> *... I firmly believe that if the whole materia medica, as now used, could be sunk to the bottom of the sea, it would be all the better for mankind — and all the worse for the fishes.*

Oliver Wendell Holmes
Medical Essays (Boston, 1883)

The U.S. medical care system is terrific in some ways, and not so good in others. It is important that you know or at least possess some guidelines to assist you in making distinctions between what it does well versus poorly or not at all. In part, the problems with the system are related to semantics. People have a tendency to refer to a health care system when, in fact, there is no such creature. More will be said of this shortly; for starters, let me summarize ten major problems of the "system" by whatever name is given to the quantity, quality, arrangement, nature, and relationships of people and resources in the provision of health care.

1. It costs too much. Prices for medical care have risen faster over the past several years than for just about any other commodity or service. The rate of rise is much greater than the inflation rate; from 1960 to 1982 the total spending as a nation for medical care jumped from $27 billion to nearly $300 billion! Costs have doubled every five years; if present trends continue, the bill will hit one trillion dollars by the year 2000. That figure, incidentally, was the total Gross National Product two years ago; so you can see that things (costs) are a bit out of control. A major reason why this is happening is that there has not been and still is no effective incentive for doctors and others within the system to control costs.

Imagine that — $300 billion! Does *anybody* sense what that means? Here is one way to render this level of investment in sickness care comprehensible.

For starters, picture a one-foot stack of one-thousand-dollar bills. That stack is worth one million dollars. It takes a million one-thousand-dollar bills to make a billion-dollar stack. Do you know how high that stack would be? The answer is 1,000 feet tall, the height of a 50-story building. Remember, this is just a one-billion-dollar pile of one-thousand-dollar bills. To stack three hundred billion dollars (using one-thousand-dollar bills), you would need 300 piles of bills, each 50 stories high.

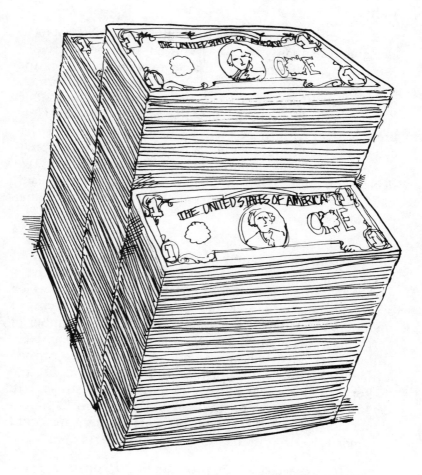

I think Congress should pass a law requiring bureaucrats to stack into neat piles the equivalent in "funny money" of what is being lavished in real dollars on sickness care. If nothing else, such a procedure would help us recall "the good old days" when a billion dollars meant something.

2. Medical services are not sufficiently accessible or available; the quality of care is uneven; treatments are discontinuous or fragmentary due to overspecialization and poor coordination of the overall system; and consumers often feel that providers of care are impersonal and aloof. An elaborate planning system has been created by Congress to deal with these issues. Unfortunately, in part because of extensive regulatory procedures and capital-expansion controls, little has been achieved in nearly two decades of quasi-governmental, quasi-"grass-roots" health planning. There is still no incentive for doctors and other providers to control costs.

3. Too many mistakes are made; surgery is often employed inappropriately, drugs are used to excess, and hospitalizations are often unnecessary. Some studies have shown that three- to four-fold variations in regional rates for six basic procedures were explainable by payment methods, availability of hospital beds, and the number of surgeons in the area (*New England Journal of Medicine*, 1969, 281: 880-84). Five billion tranquilizer pills are prescribed annually, 39 million of which were for Valium alone, the doctors' most popular remedy for "everyday" stress. Jere Goyan, FDA (Food and Drug Administration) Commissioner in 1980, stated that overmedicated Americans could cut their total drug intake in half without harm.

4. The expectations of providers and consumers are hazardous to both parties. The doctors find themselves expected to play godlike roles of healer and fixer; consumers are conditioned to be intimidated, ignorant, not responsible, and generally helpless. These role extremes have

been changing in recent years due to the influence of activist providers and consumers, but the above-noted stereotypes still exist for most people.

5. Not all drugs or medical procedures are safe or effective. Drugs are sometimes used for years, then pulled off the market when they are shown to do more harm than good. (The FDA, by the way, was set up to test for safety, not efficacy.) In 1974, 30,000 deaths were attributed to prescription drugs.* Examples of dubious though widespread surgical approaches include coronary-artery bypass, tonsillectomy, hernia operations, coronary-artery-bypass grafts, radical mastectomy, adenoidectomy, and hysterectomies, to name a few. Hospital income, unfortunately, is related to the amount of surgery performed, as is, of course, the income of surgeons. Also, in 1974 the U.S. Congress issued a report estimating that as much as 2.3 million operations were unnecessary, the costs for which were $3.9 billion and 11,000 lives lost.†

6. There is a widespread belief through the system that health education and prevention (and, therefore, any other kind of behavior-change program) does not work. Health-education programs, it is true, have not been effective, but not because poor lifestyle habits are intractable. The usual failures in prevention-type programs are related to poor program design, emphasis on negative messages, lack of imagination, information giving without active involvement and participation by clients and patients, low funding, and poor health-education role models, to name but a few.

7. Despite all the attention and resources, the medical system has not given us raised health status or longer lives. For people 65 years of age, according to the Metropolitan Life Insurance Company, life expectancy in 1970 was but

---

*James Fadiman, M.D. "Ground Rules for Integral Medicine," *Holistic Health Review*, 3, 1, (Fall 1979): p. 22.
†Ibid.

half a year greater than their age cohort counterparts in 1850 (77.9 versus 77.5). When medical historians look at the relevant data, they conclude that the major improvements in the health of the population have been due to factors other than medical care quality, availability, or anything else related to the medical system. McKeown and others have shown that modern advances in health (e.g., the decline of infectious diseases) primarily were due to environmental factors such as an increase in the food supply, a reduction in exposure to infection through control of air- and water-borne disease agents, behavior changes affecting controlled population growth, and the introduction of immunizations.

8. The system too often neglects the whole person. Much of what is being popularized today under the holistic health banner is a reaction to an overly mechanistic or biological medical focus. The latter tends to neglect psychological factors and subtle biochemical diversities, leading to uniformity in treatments, dosage levels, insufficient training for patient self-regulation, and no appreciation for the meaning inherent in certain, if not all, illnesses. Recently, a movement toward whole-person (mind/body/spirit) approaches has been growing in popularity. In holistic, integral, or vitalistic medicine, a symptom is not viewed in isolation but as a visible link in a complete and extraordinary chain. Symptoms are viewed as manifestations of, or messages concerning, the body's healing efforts. Most important, mind/body relationships are explored as part of understanding causation, as are habits and feelings. Of course, many practitioners who never heard about holistic medicine have intuitively employed these and related principles over many years, but the literature does not suggest that such humanistic perspectives reflect the mainstream of modern medical care.

9. The system is almost exclusively targeted on the treatment of disease and disability to the neglect of illness prevention and health promotion. A Surgeon General's Report on Health Promotion (*Healthy People,* 1979) received widespread attention because it put the government on record as supportive of a change in focus for the U.S. medical system. This document legitimized the disparate attempts in recent years to change the prevailing sickness and disability orientation. *Healthy People* states that future improvements in the health of the populace will only be achieved through a national commitment to prevent disease and promote health; the secretary of HEW (now the Department of Health and Human Services) called for a "second revolution in public health" to achieve this transfer of emphasis. Naturally, this is reasonable enough when you consider that more than fifty percent of all years of life lost are related to accidents, heart and respiratory disease, lung cancer, and suicide/homicide. The risk factors for such problems are highway speeds, failure to wear seat belts, alcohol abuse, sedentary living, smoking, high stress levels without management skills, poor nutrition, dangerous working environments, and so forth. For such risks, the medical systems can do little; the answers for these problems will not come from having more doctors, bigger and better hospitals, or more wondrous biomedical research breakthroughs.

The current craze to teach everybody cardio-pulmonary resuscitation (CPR) in order to "save" heart-attack victims is based on a noble enough goal, but in my opinion is terribly flawed. Courses are often taught by obese chain smokers; nothing is said about avoiding the habits that over a lifetime lead inexorably to heart failure and other degenerative diseases.

10. Medical care and health are used interchangeably, which confuses people and creates unachievable expectations. Walter McNerney, president of Blue Cross and Blue Shield Association (Chicago), said that we must stop throwing an array of technological processes and systems at lifestyle problems and stop equating more health services with better health. The organization of services, facilities, and manpower for delivering medical care is called the "health system." "Health" insurance is, in fact, sickness-care financial protection. The "health" planning movement has devoted nearly all of its attention to sickness-care facilities. Mental health centers spend almost all their resources on treatment of the psychologically troubled or disturbed.

Of course, this tampering with language occurs in other areas (e.g., toilet paper is now "facial quality tissue"), but the effect for present purposes is that it has obscured the dangerous omission of health promotion. Even the so-called National Institute of Health reflects the problem. It contains a National Heart, Lung, and Blood Institute, a Cancer Institute, and an Institute for Arthritis and Metabolic Diseases. There is no Institute for Health! Or Wellness!

All of these problems are widely recognized. Some progress has been made; further relief is on the way. I think your goal, at this point, is just to be aware of the problems and the wellness alternative. You should be quite clear about the dramatic difference in emphasis that distinguishes the wellness movement from the concerns of the health care system. The following diagram should help you get a clear picture of this varying emphasis. Think of a continuum from worseness at the bottom to wellness at the top, as indicated below.

WORSENESS/WELLNESS CONTINUUM

	whole-person excellence	
	actions and payoffs	
the wellness	personal wellness plans	
movement	conscious commitment to pursue wellness	
	knowledge of principles in 5 dimensions	
	awareness of the wellness option	
NOT SICK	"HEALTH"	NOT SICK

	risk reduction
	signs and symptoms of illness
the "health"	crisis and emergencies
care system	disabilities and disorders
	depression and resignation
	death

The medical care system (called "health" care system) functions entirely below the neutral point of health as "not sick." It is pathology-bound and focused. As a result, little or nothing is done within the medical system to encourage and support healthy lifestyles. If you want attention from the medical system, you need a medical problem, not a healthy curiosity. (While true in the past, there are changes afoot. Would you believe hospital-based wellness centers? It's true. You will read about a few of these innovative medical institutions in Part Two.)

While the medical system has little to do with health, it often does play a superb role in diagnosing, treating, and arresting states of ill health. The medical system plays an important part in the economy. It has social and political functions that are as important as its therapeutic and scientific roles. It generates products, supports suppliers, undertakes research and development, sets up financing mechanisms for capital formation and cash-flow purposes, creates markets for insurance, and otherwise connects with and supports an elaborate service society.

It is possible to be aware of the problems with the system while still acknowledging and making use of its strengths. For example, modern medicine is often superbly effective. And, it does more than help people to get back to a state of non-illness. It provides a source of comfort, justification, explanation, and reassurance.

Here are a few guidelines to consider in terms of what to expect and how to deal with the medical system for those occasions when you slip below the non-sick level on the continuum.

- Do not confuse positive health and good medical care. The latter is important but does not lead to the former.
- Only you can be responsible for your medical care. Never delegate final decision making and accountability for assessing alternatives and taking action.
- Become aware on medical issues. Read the recommended books in the resource guide (Part Three) and pursue added knowledge in areas of particular interest. A medical self-care capability can be both invaluable and economical.
- Explore alternatives and options before consenting to surgery or drug treatments. Get second opinions.* Remember that a diagnosis is not as important as the course of action contemplated; the risks in the latter are what deserve most of your attention.
- Know that most illnesses are self-limiting. Not every malady either has or needs a cure.

---

*Be careful, however. When Rodney Dangerfield was told by his doctor that he was overweight, he said: "I don't trust your judgement. I want a second opinion." His doctor said, "OK, you're ugly."

- There are no villains. The ten problems sketched above are not evidence of a plot against the laity by a privileged group or groups of professionals. Things just developed that way over time for many reasons, only a few of which are fully grasped. Awareness is adequate; placing blame is a waste of energy and inherently unfair.
- Realize that symptoms usually mean something. Try to develop your skills in interpreting messages from your "inner" self.

Maybe there will be major improvements in the medical system in the years to come. Such changes would certainly be welcomed by the system's friends and critics alike. In the meantime, however, be aware of the situation as it is. Do the many things you can to make the best of any illness condition through knowledge and personal control.

This overview completes Day Three. Thanks for working your way through this. You are now in a good position to move on, tomorrow, to the next step. Make a check at the back for completing today's lesson.

By the way, it is not true that Californians are like granola. That is, if you remove the nuts and fruits, you are still left with lots of flakes.

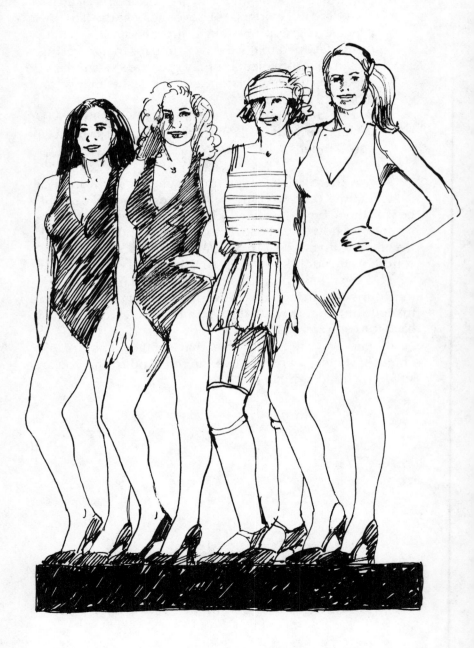

Day Four

Take An Inventory Of Cultural Norms: Many Are Hazardous To Your Health

Purpose: To make you consciously aware of the influences exerted by social expectations and unwritten rules. Also, to look at the dynamics of norms in choosing and maintaining lifestyle patterns for health enhancement.

A society is in jeopardy if a member of that society must be a fool, a martyr, or a hero to do what is right.
—Plato

Given encouragement and support, I believe everyone would choose life purposes and habits that enable extraordinary levels of individual and societal wellness. Similarly, given another kind of encouragement and support, everyone would have low self-esteem, a poor self-concept, a rotten diet, a bad attitude toward exercise, high stress levels, a tendency to blame others rather than to take responsibility, and all the other characteristics of a worseness lifestyle.

Wellness is not a condition of special virtue or superior

will power, higher morality, or divine selection. Wellness is, in my view, a reflection of cultural norms, which include the uncountable influences (some direct but mostly not so) which guide and reinforce attitude and behavior choices.

Those of us who enjoy a wellness lifestyle do so primarily because we stumbled into or otherwise got ourselves exposed to basically favorable environments at opportune times. Few of us are heroes, fools, or martyrs — we just have "head-start" cultures acting upon us that make wellness more likely. We are the fortunate few who, despite the fact that the larger society is oriented below the not-sick line, came to perceive that there is a direction for health above that line. It is called wellness, and a big part of it is learning to identify and shape the many cultures of which we are a part. This is the subject of Day Four.

Health education and traditional prevention programs have focused upon individual behavior to the neglect of the environment in which such behavior takes place. In pursuing wellness, you will have at least three advantages going for you that are lacking in traditional efforts to make changes: (1) your motivation will be based on positive expectations; (2) the specific activities (e.g., relaxation exercises, different food choices, etc.) will be integrated in a balanced approach, so that change in one dimension complements another; and (3) deliberate efforts will be made to understand the unwritten but powerful codes that affect efforts to maintain lifestyle change.

Have you noticed that it is easier to take better care of yourself in some settings than in others? Can you think of instances when you had not intended to do one thing or another but, to go along with the group, found yourself joining in? Chances are good that this happens every day. All of us belong to a variety of cultures, which are simply groups of people who come together, deliberately or otherwise, and in so doing influence each other's ideas and behaviors. Social scientists call these influences "norms." Norms are standards and expectations, and there are so many norms in your life that you are probably not even consciously aware of but a small number of them. Norms affect how you dress, talk, eat, work, and so on. They influence what you like or dislike. Norms are essential for all groups — without them there would be chaos. The issue is not whether to have norms, but rather to understand and to choose the norms that support you. Yet, with few exceptions, you never got to choose the norms you now live with. They just seemed to come with everything else, as culturally agreed upon perspectives. Nothing could seem more natural. Norms represent "the way things always have been around here." In pursuing a wellness lifestyle, it makes good sense at the start to think about the norms in cultures of which you are a part.

You belong, as does everyone else, to a variety of cultures and subcultures. Cultures are groups of people with shared histories. The family, for example, is a culture. So are all the varied groups of which you are a member, including your associates at work or school, your neighborhood, church, friends, clubs, and so on. These cultures, and the subcultures within them, are usually loaded with norms which work against positive health. Norms, standard attitudes or behaviors that are expected, supported and reinforced by members of the culture, are pervasive. Not all norms are rationally chosen or are a part of the conscious awareness of the members of the cultures that sustain them, but they are powerful influences nonetheless. They represent "the way things are" or the notion that "we have always done it this way."

It is extremely difficult for one who is not addicted to a wellness lifestyle to initiate meaningful habit changes and to sustain a health-enriching pattern of living without awareness of and safeguards against adverse health norms. A lineup of cultures and subcultures steeped in norms that inhibit wellness is awfully hard to overcome. For this reason, it is always easier to start a healthy behavior than to follow through with it and to make it a valued part of your life. You could say there are two kinds of health initiatives: short-term and long-term. The latter are feasible only when the norms of the culture are conducive to wellness — unless you are a hero and can overcome the pressures of peers, institutions, and traditions to conform to customary practices which are decidedly unhealthy. Even when you hold views at variance with the predominant norms, the pressures, temptations, and opportunities of the non-supportive environment make it difficult to resist "going along."

Think about the messages, customs, expectations, and reinforcements of your own cultures. Is it "normal," for example, to expect:

- To wake up groggy, tired, and sore?
- To stumble off to the bathroom without pause for any ritual, ceremony, or reflection on the splendor of the morning or what joyful returns could be in store for you this day?
- To have ham, bacon, sausage, eggs, donuts, and/or similar high-fat foods for breakfast?
- To experience a freeway commute in a fuel-inefficient automobile in a stressful rush to an office or school?
- To take coffee breaks throughout the day?
- To have alcohol with lunch?
- To mix business with food, or to eat while engaged in other activities?
- To repeat the breakfast pattern of large amounts of saturated fats, in addition to high levels of sugar, sodium, cholesterol, and varied additives in your processed lunch?
- To have smoke in the air you breathe?
- To accept the notion that an exercise routine during business hours would not be appropriate?
- To accept more responsibility than you can reasonably manage?
- To work later than regular hours on a frequent basis,

and to carry work home with you?
- To return home tired and frustrated, uninterested in play, exercise, or fun and games?
- To prepare or be served food without an equal regard for nutritive value as for taste?
- To spend hours smoking, drinking, and watching television?
- To retire without having some period of reflection and/or celebration?

You may have good intentions, but the influences of the culture that get in the way often seem overwhelming. Too often, the worseness norms are more than you can withstand, in the long run. You then blame yourself for lack of will power, discipline, and self-responsibility; but in a subtle way you have been overpowered by the nonsupportive environment in which you are living.

The cultures we live with are loaded with norms that complicate healthful lifestyles. At every level, worseness norms adversely affect our prospects for the successful pursuit of wellness practices. The norms that predominate are those which discourage exercise, encourage food practices and sedentary lifestyles leading to obesity and dissolution, promote ghastly habits (e.g., smoking and substance abuse), support low expectations for positive health and human potential, and suggest that a dependence on doctors and drugs is a reasonable point of view. In short, it is not an exaggeration to state that our illness-inducing cultures wreak more havoc with the health of Americans than all the Commie plots, iatrogenic (disease-causing) doctors, tse-tse flies, and things-that-go-bump-in-the-night put together. Cultures are powerful!

Most norms, of course, such as the way we dress, do not make any difference one way or another to our health. A few, however, have important consequences, affecting not only illness levels (of some consequence, to be sure) but, most significantly, the quality of our experience and level of aliveness.

Norms can be more powerful than intentions and resolutions, if their power is not understood and taken into account. Many have found, for example, that it is easier to buy jogging shoes than it is to find the time, encouragement, and support system needed in order to wear them out.

In a culture that supported wellness, you would not have to contend with:

- School and office cafeterias, airports, and other public places that offer devitalized, highly processed and refined meals.
- Expectations that cars should be used to travel even short distances.
- Advertisements that portray smoking, alcohol and caffeine consumption, drug taking, and other forms of self-abuse as fashionable, hip, and desirable.
- Norms that suggest that poor physical conditioning is socially acceptable, understandable, and to be expected as people get older.
- Doctors, hospitals, health-insurance programs, and other health-system influences that are set up and oriented to illness treatment to the neglect of health promotion and which fail to help people cope with negative health cultures.
- High stress levels in job situations without meditation periods and group-relaxation sessions built into the normal routine.
- Reward systems that employ rich foods such as ice creams, pies, cakes and the rest in association with celebrations.
- Customs that lead us to associate having a good time, relaxing, and enjoyable social relations with overeating, alcohol abuse, smoking, and other health-reducing activities.
- An economic and social system that supports waste, high-fat and high-sugar diets, the availability of guns,

the absence of mandatory helmet wearing by motorcyclists, and similar policies that raise death and morbidity rates.

· A subculture that gives respect to persons who claim they can consume and tolerate large amounts of alcohol and engage in recreational forms of substance abuse.

· A television industry that permits commercials for sugared cereals, candy bars, packaged candies, cakes and cookies to be directed at children.

· An understanding that it is really OK to drive over fifty-five miles per hour and not wear seat belts.

· The notion that men should not express feelings, be gentle, embrace other men, or otherwise express tenderness.

· The belief that women should not be aggressive, career-oriented, unattached, childless, or otherwise able to function in "masculine" forms, should they desire these options.

· The high social costs of large numbers of distressed individuals who have worked so hard that they've lost contact with other parts of their existence, such as children, avocations, causes, friendships, and so on.

· Educational materials and messages from parents, doctors, and other authorities that emphasize over and over the details relating to minimal requirements for non-illness, and offer no insights regarding optimal well-being.

· Omnipresent vending machines, "good humor" pushers, and other entrapments to impulse buying of sugary junk products.

These customs and established influences cannot be taken lightly. You generate a lot of resistance if you disregard a norm. Exercise is not highly valued in most groups; minimizing exertion is. Try an experiment if you ever have a chance to drive a group of people to work or children to school. Without discussing it, park a mile from your destination and announce that an opportunity to stretch the legs and warm the cardiovascular system is being provided. Note the level of enthusiasm this evokes. Or, dress differently from the custom, or sit in someone else's place, or eat in a "strange" manner. All such behaviors will generate a lot of attention, because you will be acting at variance with the norms regarding how people are supposed to act in these situations.

Norms that support worseness are built into our cultures through family life, jobs, institutions, and the medical system. Though we prize freedom in this country, we are not truly free if we are controlled by norms of which we are only dimly aware.

A COURSE OF ACTION

Forget about becoming a martyr, a fool, or a hero in order to overcome the adverse norms of the many cultures and subcultures of which you are a part. It takes too much energy to be a hero, and the other choices are not very appealing to anyone like yourself with a wellness orientation. For the limited purpose of this Day's program, which is simple but critical awareness, there are but a few things to keep in mind.

For starters, simply be aware that norms are changeable, and that some norms change rather remarkably over time. Consider that, just four centuries ago, it was the norm to believe that the Earth was flat and that the Sun revolved around us rather than the reverse. Everybody believed that. If you took a contrary position, you were thought very strange. Pressures were brought to bear on Galileo and others to get in line with the beliefs that were part of that cultural system. Just a little over 100 years ago, it was a cultural norm in some parts of this country to believe that slavery was a necessary social and economic institution, and a part of the natural order of things. Norms and "God's way" are often closely connected. Until 1903, it was the norm to believe that man would never fly — if you thought otherwise, you were considered pretty weird. Until the late 1920s, the norm was that women should not vote, or we would really screw up the society (some still hold to this norm). Until 1954, there was a norm that man could not run a mile in less than four minutes (more than a thousand such miles have been run since). Other examples of norm changes could be cited (e.g., man on the moon), but you get the idea. You can change the nature and thus the effects of the cultures and norms that affect your commitment to and performance of a wellness lifestyle. In doing so, you can realize norm changes more dramatic for you than the examples just given.

One of the cultural norms that most inhibits lifestyle excellence, in my view, is the pervasive agreement throughout the medical system and the larger society that people are healthy if they are not sick. The absence of disease, illness, injury, and other debilitations is seen as the predominant health goal, and this objective is reinforced throughout the system. That was the point of the Worseness/Wellness Continuum. You can begin the process of shaping a supportive environment by reaffirming your commitment to a far higher standard of well-being than simply meeting minimal requirements for non-illness.

In rejecting the prevailing norm that non-illness equals health, you put yourself in a position to begin a systematic process of personally led cultural change. This will do more for your health than national health insurance, unlimited drugs, or a doctor in your bedroom and a season pass to the hospital of your choice.

In addition to being changeable, norms are also recognizable, if you choose to pay attention. Naturally, this takes a bit of discipline at first. After all, we have been programmed for many years to "go along, that is the way we have always done things around here." If we live in an illness culture that is essentially not set up to support and promote optimal health, which I believe is the reality of our society, then we have to pay attention on an individual basis to separate those norms which aid from those that get in the way of wellness living.

Among the changeable, norm-shaping influences that clearly get in the way of wellness lifestyles are media messages. Alcohol and tobacco advertising pervade the society through hundreds of millions of advertising dollars spent each year by manufacturers of both products to equate in our minds the use of alcohol and tobacco with the good, healthy, and happy life.

Another cultural enemy or adverse norm to be acknowledged and then combatted in varied ways is television. Recent studies* show that the average American family spends 6½ hours per day in front of the tube. Ever wonder what kinds of norms are transmitted to the populace via this powerful medium? Here is a summary of a few:

- Society is a man's world of action, power, and danger.
- Crime is pervasive (while frighteningly high in the real world, it is 10 times more so on TV; there are 5 acts of violence per hour during prime time, 18 such acts per hour during children's weekend viewing hours).
- Pain, suffering, sickness, injury, and medical help are the most popular topics of conversation.
- On daytime serials, the hit parade of occurrences are psychiatric disorders, heart attacks, pregnancies, automobile accidents, attempted homicides, attempted suicides, and diseases (infectious), in that order.
- Daytime serials are the greatest single source of medical advice in America.

---

*George Gerbner et al., "Programming Health Portrayals: What Viewers See, Say, and Do" prepared for *Television and Behavior: Ten Years of Scientific Progress and Implications for the 80s,* the National Institute of Mental Health update of the original report of the Surgeon General's Scientific Advisory Committee on Television and Social Behavior. (University of Pennsylvania, January 1981).

- The average child sees about 22,000 commercials; young children often cannot differentiate between programs and commercials.
- More than half the food-product commercials are for junk-food items (high calorie, high sugar).
- Most such advertising is for sugared cereals, candy bars, and other sweets presented as between-meal snacks.
- Ninety percent of all obese people on TV are black (a figure disproportionate to their representation in the U.S. population).
- Incidences of characters refusing to smoke or expressing antismoking sentiments are rare; the same is true of drinking behaviors.

And so it goes, as Kurt Vonnegut might write. The authors of the report suggest that television dominates the attention of the least educated and poorest segments of our population, the people who have least access to needed information about nutrition and other wellness dimensions. The norms, in other words, are not serving these cultural groups. Individual action in the face of social pressures and the kinds of beliefs perpetrated by this kind of TV will be difficult, to put it mildly.

TV is another reason why the norms of the many cultures of which we are all a part must be taken very seriously, identified by those affected, and discussed in the sense of making conscious change, where necessary.

So, this is it for Day Four. Begin to think in these terms and distinguish supportive from inhibitory influences all around you.

Einstein was once asked, "What is the most important question facing human beings?"

He said, "The question is this: Is the Universe friendly?"

You do well to ask yourself the same question with slight modification. That is, is the culture (or cultures) of which you are a part friendly to the kind of lifestyle you have selected, or do you have to go out of your way to pursue the heights?

An awareness about the power of norms will serve you well. For now, give yourself credit for another day of relentless progress toward a wellness lifestyle. Check Day Four as complete.

(Know how many psychiatrists it takes to change a light bulb? Just one, but the bulb has to want to change.)

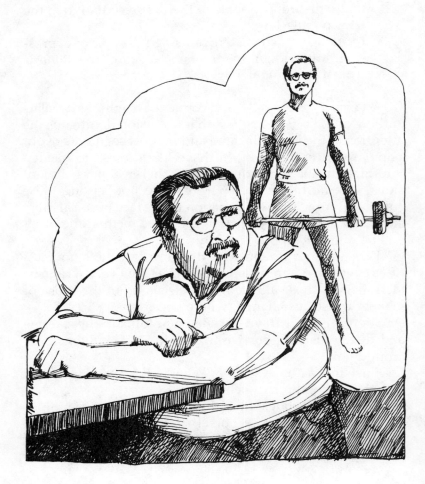

Day Five

Draw A Picture Or Image Of What It Means To Be A Healthy Person

Purpose: To raise your level of curiosity about the end results of a lifelong pursuit of wellness and to encourage you to develop a conscious awareness of what it means to be a truly healthy person.

There are many pathways to whole-person excellence, but your chances of arriving without undue frustrations, detours, and dead ends are greater with a map of the territory. The "map" in this case is a clear set of mental pictures of what wellness looks like, how it feels, how things are for those who live this way, and similar unmistakable characteristics associated with optimal health. You have had plenty of exposure to illness states. Though you never selected this specialization (unless you are a physician), you have been trained over the years as an expert in *negative* health. You learned as a child the names of scores of diseases, heard about people who experienced one or more of these debilitations, and learned to memorize half a dozen or more "warning signs" of heart attacks, cancer, and so forth. You have, no doubt, heard of cardio-pulmonary-resuscitation (CPR) courses or *minimum* daily requirements for vitamins? Nearly everybody is acquainted

with these and other important facts about death prevention and illness avoidance. But how many of us have been
taught about or have been given chances to investigate the
other side of the Worseness/Wellness Continuum? Very
few. The U.S. government spent billions in recent years
developing profiles of illness and otherwise assessing, class-
ifying, and defining non-health — and not a penny investi-
gating what positive health is all about. How many times
have we read about studies which suggest that ten percent
of the population suffers from mental illness, that the annual cost of such illness is more than $21 billion dollars, that
alcoholism each year costs the nation another $15 billion,
that drug abuse adds another $10 billion, and so on for all
the downside repercussions of worseness conditions? Often, no doubt. Have you ever read a report about how
healthy people live in our society, how they developed their
life styles, and why they maintain such practices? Probably
never — if you have, please send me a copy; I'd love to see it.
Due to this lack of interest, about all the government knows
about a healthy person is that he or she is one who has been
inadequately studied. This leaves something to be desired!

One challenge you face in overcoming negative health
norms and acting in such a way as to enjoy advancing
toward your best possibilities along your own special paths
to excellence is to learn about *positive* health. Create a clear
perception of what superhealth will mean in your life. How
will things be different? What will you do that you do not do
now? The sharper your pictures and higher your expectations, the more likely and ambitious your realizations will
become.

In order to develop your own set of expectations and
mental pictures of what specific results to expect from a
wellness lifestyle, become aware of the general characteristics of healthy people. You will not find much on this
subject in the medical literature, but the humanistic
psychologists have had a lot to say on the subject. What
follows are images of optimal health based in part on the

writings of Abraham Maslow and Carl Rogers, and in part on a few of my own ideas. Naturally, few people have all these characteristics going for them, but fortunately, this is unnecessary in order to enjoy wellness! Just take what applies and shape the material to fit into your purposes and perspectives. The key, when you get right to the "bottom line," is to have an unmistakable set of mind images or pictures of what wellness means and encompasses *in your life*. Whether "traveling hopefully" (which Parkinson suggested is better than to arrive) or simply maintaining an established wellness lifestyle, it helps to know as much as possible about the values you treasure. Here, then, is a partial summary of positive health values which I believe are worth working for and safeguarding when achieved. Each should be useful to you in shaping your own wellness goals and positive health images. They are not definitions — just images of positive states of whole-person being for you to work with in shaping your own expectations!

 • High self-esteem and a positive outlook. This characteristic encompasses a favorable self-image and a deep-seated respect for who you are. It means your self-esteem is not on the line every time you encounter new challenges, tests, or difficulties. You can screw up royally, on occasion, and not diminish yourself. You genuinely are pleased with what you represent, and your general orientation is that life gets better as you continue to evolve. An expansive self-image and outlook makes the future more attractive — it is a mental blueprint that makes the unknown seem non-threatening, even alluring.
 • A foundation philosophy and sense of purpose. This means that you have worked out and are comfortable with a meaning or significance to your existence. You may not have discovered "the answer(s)" for anyone else, but you have quiet confidence in a working set of informal hypotheses that guide your actions and help you interpret what your life is all about. Your sense of purpose and philosophy

provide a spiritual (ethical) and practical grounding for all the details, decisions, circumstances, and events that affect your existence — and a channel for most of life's energies.

· Self-responsible and self-aware. Some of the ideas associated with this characteristic are an awareness of your current values, needs, strengths, images, and limitations, an ability to learn from events and improve, and a capacity to regulate your behavior in accordance with your own standards. To be self-responsible is to be, in part, autonomous, intrinsically self-governing, and relatively free of unexamined personal beliefs, group norms, and pressures which inhibit potentials. A healthy person is inner directed, believes that he/she is responsible for illness and health, success and failure, and just about everything else. They are more often the cause, not the effect, of what happens to and around them.

· Humor, happiness and joy. You do not have to be funny to have a sense of humor, nor do you feel a need to practice the art at the expense of others. This characteristic involves an ability to laugh at and appreciate the absurd in yourself and in events around you. (If you cannot laugh at yourself on occasion, maybe you are not in on the joke.) No one ever has or probably ever will define humor, happiness or joy with universal acceptance, and it is unnecessary in any event. One totally unscientific but possibly useful indicator of how you are doing in this regard is to look at yourself a lot. Not in the mirror — that is usually rehearsed. I mean, tune in to your facial expression and feeling states as you walk about, or while you sit at a desk or work on a job and so on. These are pretty good guides. If you catch yourself frowning, grimacing, being scared, tense, and down in the mouth (and navel), it could be you need to work on raising your humor, happiness and joy quotient. You may have rectum retinitis and not even know it (i.e., a nasty condition caused by the crossing of the optic nerves with the anal neurons, leading to a crappy outlook on things). This is not inherited — you can *choose* to learn ways to be happier and more open to fun and peak moments in your life.

· Support and concern for others and the environment. Healthy people grow and flourish from their activities and the way they participate in life. They grow from contributing. In addition to a human support network interested in wellness, they believe it is crucial to be on appreciative terms with Mother Nature. Personally, I think we should all seek out at least three awes per day of wonderment at the splendor of the Earth and Cosmos (without neglecting the daisies, dolphins, whales, beasties, and so forth). In short, an ecological consciousness seems a vital element in a healthy person's makeup, encompassing a respect for the interconnectedness of all things. It includes an awareness of and concern about physical and psychological pollutants (sexism, racism, ageism), social oppression (poverty), global hazards (war), and similar matters beyond the neighborhood.

· Conscious commitment to well-being and excellence. This characteristic derives from a decision to go first class in life, a strong motivation to expand, and a dedication to heights of consequence and distinction. The unwillingness to settle for mediocrity or getting by is expressed in high levels of competence in work and play. A conscious choice to go for your potentials entails full use of talents and the exercise of creativity with minimal inhibitions. It is not likely that you would long sustain a wellness lifestyle without a conscious recognition that this was a choice you made and intended to achieve.

· Sense of balance and an integrated lifestyle. A unifying outlook, an avoidance of extremes, and a tolerance for ambiguity are parts of this characteristic. An ability to function effectively in the midst of complexity, to be able to manage in varied situations wherein "rights" conflict, and to display interpersonal skills are also facets of this optimally well characteristic.

· Freedom from low-level worseness addictions. In his

famous "hierarchy of needs," Maslow* argued that security, safety, support, and other needs had to be attended before self-actualization and personal transformation were possible. So it is with a wellness lifestyle, the pursuit of excellence, and the realization of characteristics associated with living at the heights of your potentials. If you are free of negative addictions, you are relieved of burdens that otherwise wear you down and distract from the positive side of the continuum.

· Capacity to cope and to learn. "Superhealthy" people do well under duress; they cope effectively, they adapt, and they learn from experience. They see crises as opportunities for growth and new directions. They expect change and make the best of it. Change sometimes seems for the better, sometimes not. We all have our seasons. You cannot change the weather, but you can locate yourself in certain psychological climates that are more hospitable than others. Pay attention to how you respond under pressure, frustration, uncertainty, and hardship. Even if you "blow it," simply consider the situation, think about ways to better manage such situations next time, and get on with it. There is no profit in dumping on yourself for what you might have done or said, but there is considerable value in using such episodes for self-appraisal and redirection.

· Grounded in reality. This means that you can see things as they are, not as you would like them to be. There is much to be said for seeing the world through rose-colored glasses, but you should know when to remove them. It is an art worth cultivating to be able to spot mountebanks, fakirs, and holistic charlatans. Cultivate a respect for evidence. Amid conflicting claims and massive data in the health field and other areas of life, a discerning mind, able to evaluate and decide, is another crucial characteristic of the healthy "whole" person. It surely entails an abiding suspicion of those who claim a pipeline to or possession of

---

*Abraham H. Maslow, *The Farther Reaches of Human Nature* (New York: Viking Press, 1971).

"ultimate truths," for such claimants have an uncomfortable propensity to talk about "final solutions." As Dr. William Hettler has often mentioned: "There are no simple solutions — there are only intelligent choices."

· Highly conditioned and physically fit. While optimal physical well-being is just one of the purposes and elements of a wellness lifestyle, it is an important area that leads to gains in the mental and emotional spheres. When you show high performance on the physical vital signs, you are on your way to achieving all the rest. The three keys are endurance, strength, and flexibility. (Vital signs and the elements of fitness are the subjects of Days 12 and 7, respectively.)

· A capacity to love and a willingness to be nurtured. The truly healthy person has deep roots of connectedness, and places a major priority on close relationships with others. Peak experiences seem higher when shared.

· Viable in the world. The healthy person manages his/her resources appropriately and produces results that have an impact of consequence.

· Effective communications. A capability to make yourself understood in a wide range of circumstances, and to appreciate and recognize the meanings in other people's words and behaviors, is a valued component of the genuinely well individual. Relationships work best when you can deal with difficult points of view at home, the workplace, and in other situations.

· Integrity. A healthy person lives with and up to his/her standards. These measures for judgment are not compromised for temporary advantage; on the contrary, they are a source of strength *and* advantage.

There are many additional phrases, concepts, ideas, and terms that could be discussed in the context of states of positive health. The major purpose of this Fifth Day is to help you prepare to sharpen your own image of what high-level wellness can look, feel, and be like for you.

The steady pursuit of these states of well-being is of far greater consequence to your lifestyle efforts than any specific courses of action you might take to achieve them. Thus, go easy on yourself when you do not do what you believe you should (e.g., exercise every day) or do what you should not (e.g., eat junk food). The course of action is just a detail; the goal of true value is the overall familiarity with, and commitment to, such characteristics as described above.

One final word on these pictures of optimal health. Remember that *you* determine *what health can be* and *when you get there*. Novelist Kurt Vonnegut, Jr., wrote a book (*Mother Night*) about a double agent who crossed over and became a triple spy, then switched a few more times, and forgot which side he was on. The moral was: "You are what you pretend to be — you must be very careful what you pretend to be." You be careful too — do not settle for anything less than the magnificence that is within you. By setting a higher standard, by "pretending" to be as much as you can be, by raising your expectations, you will invariably magnify your results.

Please take another look at the preceding images of healthy functioning and make a list in your own words of those characteristics which you think are important as guides in your own growth and development. Add phrases that you think are important. When you feel satisfied with your list as a temporary statement of your healthy pictures and images, simply write on the paper next to each characteristic what percentage of this state you already manifest, and where you expect to be next year at this time. For example, if you marked self-responsible and self-aware and decided that you were at the 50-percent level of mastery, your one-year target might be at 80 percent, and so on for each characteristic. The idea for writing out assessments and desired directions is to strengthen yourself psychologically for awareness and action purposes.

Sometimes it takes a special effort to convince yourself

that you truly have all the qualities needed to be a well person. At a conscious level, you may want to believe these things about yourself (which then makes it possible to live accordingly), but "deep down" you are skeptical at best and downright unconvinced at worst. If this is the case, and even if it is not, you may want to employ a few affirmations or self-statements about how terrific you really are.

Here are a few developed by the staff of the North Cascade Wellness Institute (described in Part Two) that touch on many of the characteristics of being a healthy person.

AFFIRMATIONS FOR A WELLNESS LIFESTYLE

High Self-Esteem

I am a capable person and I delight in solving a challenging problem.

I enjoy spending time with myself as I am my own best advisor.

Sense of Purpose

I know where I am going and I enjoy the accomplishment of each step.

I am needed by others and love being there to lend my support.

Acceptance of Self and Others

I am a sensitive, caring person and express my feelings openly to those important in my life.

I am in this world and so are you, together we will make it our own Utopia.

Peak Experiences

I cherish all of the unforgettable times I have spent loving and sharing time with the people who are close to me and touch my life.

I have an incredible supply of energy and this allows me to reach peak performance levels consistently.

Integrity (Competence)

I am honest with myself and, therefore, all others.

I am an excellent teacher — logical, well-prepared, and completely at ease.

I am well-organized in every phase of my life.

Democratic Personality

I respect the opinions of those who see things differently than I do.

No one in the world is more or less important than I.

Creativity and Sense of Humor

I surround myself with people who have a twinkle in their eye and a smile on their face; a good laugh is revitalizing.

I have a constant flow of creative and unique ideas.

Affectionate and Expressive

I constantly develop feelings of self-respect and high self-esteem in myself and in others.

I have a warm, loving, affectionate home.

Commitment to Excellence

My goals are high and I reach them easily.

Those of us who work together constantly express our commitment to excellence through actions as well as attitudes.

Infrequent Illness

Because I live using wellness concepts, I am seldom ill.

Life is glorious and I use every minute before it disappears.

I have no time for illness.

Free of Negative Addiction

I live my life in a sea of positive concepts.

I enjoy my positive addictions and the impact they have on my life. I have no room for negative addictions.

High Level of Fitness

I am lean, mean, and sexy and rejoice in the feeling.

I am in super condition and I love the feeling of strength that follows my daily workout.

I, and I alone, am responsible for my high-level wellness. I am overjoyed by the impact my own strength commitment has on my quality of life.*

You are making wonderful progress. Give yourself a pat on the back, and a rub on the tummy for good measure. You deserve it, but even if you did not it would be a good idea to pause for a little self-acknowledgment now and throughout the day — every day. After all, is this not just another part of your picture of what it means to be a healthy person?

(Do you know what is the leading cause of death for rats in North American medical centers? The answer is on the bottom of the page, upside down.)

Good show, my friend. Mark Day Five complete.

---

*The contributions of Ron Worley, Julie Bloomfield, Jill Wolfe, Kathy Herron, Angela Lester, and Debbie Miller of the North Cascade Wellness Institute are gratefully acknowledged.

Answer to above question: Research!

IT'S GOOD TO KNOW THAT,
IF I BEHAVE STRANGELY ENOUGH,

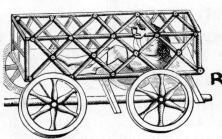

SOCIETY
WILL TAKE
FULL
RESPONSIBILITY
FOR ME.

Ashleigh
Brilliant

Day Six

Begin Work On Your Black Belt In Self-Responsibility

Purpose: To persuade you to adopt an "exaggerated" perspective on personal responsibility and to acquaint you with several important considerations about accountability in a wellness philosophy.

THE STATUS QUO AND A FEW PERSPECTIVES

Ashleigh Brilliant's cartoon "Potshot" sums up what might be the great "unknown" number one health problem in the U.S. today — lack of incentives or public education for taking personal responsibility. Hundreds of millions of North Americans are not aware that they are primarily accountable for their own health status and the ultimate fate of their lives. It is no accident that the condition exists: it is a predictable consequence of unplanned health policies. These policies are constructed on the unwritten, unspoken, and largely unrecognized but nonetheless pernicious reality that we are nearly all dependent souls, unable or at least unwilling to account for our own destinies — and to organize our lives accordingly.

Think of how the system works, as described in Day Three: health insurance pays *only* for sickness care; doctors are trained *only* to treat illness, and thus most know little about wellness; and government supports *only* medical system planning and a miniscule level of risk-reduction activity under the deceptive banner of health promotion. This flight from self-responsibility is most revealed in U.S. national health-insurance plans which, in paying for unlimited sickness care without regard for causation, while at the same time including no benefits or programs for health enhancement, unwittingly reward *delegation* and penalize *accountability*. In other words, people who take initiatives to stay fit, manage stress, create supportive environments, and otherwise pursue wellness would pay more under national health-insurance schemes because their taxes would be used to subsidize the masses doing nothing for themselves. Critics of this system, the few who urge greater attention to programs that promote accountability and incentives for health-enrichment practices are accused of "victim blaming," of not having sufficient compassion for the unfortunates who are only pawns in a world not of their own devising.

I mention all this at the start in order that you have a feel for the broader implications of highly skilled, uncompromising, or what I call "black belt" adherence to the full spirit of the self-responsibility dimension. To put it gently, the ultimate effects of widespread adoption of the ethic of personal accountability would be far-reaching throughout our society.

The skills you cultivate, the regimen you follow, and the satisfactions you derive in each of the other four wellness dimensions are directly related to your conscious, and especially your unconscious, beliefs about the role you exert in effecting your own fate. The goal of Day Six, therefore, is to encourage and support you to persuade yourself to the deepest levels of your existence that you wield the power, the opportunity, and the absolute right to manage and direct your own fate and destiny. Being the sovereign for your fate should be seen as a joyful reality — more a gift than a burden. I believe it is in your interest to adopt this position and apply the consequences throughout this and every remaining day of your life. You will then become the cause, not the effect, of everything that happens.

By the end of this day, I hope to convince you to reconsider and reinterpret the old saw about "there but for the grace of God go I." The revisionist position that I recommend is: "Here, thanks to me, am I." The wellness slogan!

Taking responsibility for your health means making a conscious commitment to your well-being. It involves a recognition that you choose a positive existence for the pursuit of excellence affecting all four aspects of being — the physical, mental, emotional, and spiritual realms. This kind of commitment to a wellness lifestyle goes beyond goals, self-imposed disciplines, and adherence to standardized rules; self-responsibility for a wellness lifestyle transcends agreements and rules. A conscious choice for a "whole-person" pursuit of your highest potentials represents a commitment to always create the most successful existence within your reach. The nature of your approach to self-responsibility will, of course, be affected by your individual preferences, cultures, environments, and all other circumstances not always under your control. You simply do what you can about those things that can be affected, and adjust or accommodate yourself to the rest in a way that serves you to the maximum extent. Part of wellness in general and self-responsibility in particular is to become skilled at recognizing the difference.

Given the central role of self-responsibility for health, you would think that high school and college course work would be weighted toward the subject, that books would be written on the topic, that it would be part of medical self-care and first-aid courses, and that the doctors and hospital staffs would be well prepared to talk about specific applications of this basic ethic. Not so — few source materials of any kind are available and the issues surrounding personal responsibility for health are seldom adequately defined and discussed. This is unfortunate, in part because forms for self-responsibility could be a fascinating subject area to explore in otherwise dull health-education courses, and in part because it is difficult to imagine a health-education endeavor succeeding if the students are not persuaded to adopt a viewpoint of personal sovereignty for their own health.

There are two major problems that show up when surveys are taken of population attitudes toward and knowledge of health skills. One is that almost all people have a vastly exaggerated notion of the powers of medical science to restore health once it is lost — an estimation that doctors claim is grossly inaccurate and out of line with the state of the medical art and science. The other problem is that many people seem to have a belief in their own invulnerability to illness risks inherent in alcohol abuse and tobacco use. That is, a smoker will acknowledge that his/her habit is dangerous, but that he/she can somehow do it with impunity. Many people, in other words, deny self-responsibility by kidding themselves into thinking that they are charmed, immune from risks that others face, and somehow on the far right side of the bell-shaped curve. This, of course, is suicidal — but a clear manifestation of what self-responsibility is not. There seems to be an inverse correlation between a strong sense of personal responsibility and a belief in medical miracles. Unfortunately, as Bloomfield has suggested, the only place you can find omnipotent doctors is on television.

I recall a cartoon depiction of a little boy watching a man chisel on a large rock. The boy watched patiently for hours as the artist chipped away. In the last frame, as the form emerged from the rock, the boy's expression came alive and he happily exclaimed: "Wow — how did you know there was a lion in there?"

To suggest that self-responsibility is the "tool" you need to shape your own sculpture, a few additional perspectives on the idea may be in order.

Ivan Illich, in *Medical Nemesis* (Pantheon Books, 1977), claims that we have lost the capacity for self-care, that health has been medicalized, that we have become a patient population, and that we lack the rudimentary characteristics of a responsible nation with respect to our health. A strong indictment, right? Guess who Illich "credits" for the existence of this sorry state of national worseness? Not the people themselves for allowing it (assuming the judgment is valid), but rather the medical profession! Illich's reasons for blaming the doctors are interesting and you may want to read his book (reviewed on the honor roll of *High Level Wellness*). Personally, I think Illich is off target for two reasons: (1) all the iatrogenesis, or doctor-caused illness, is benign in comparison with the malpractice and poor treatment which people foist upon themselves through destructive lifestyles; and (2) blaming doctors serves no one — it is another end run around self-responsibility. If you, for example, have been encouraged to think of yourself as a patient, to think of health only in medical terms, and to think that you need a doctor's OK to pursue wellness in an integrated fashion, then that is only the way things have been up to now. You can change all that. You can decide to take back the ultimate accountability for your own well-being. Hours, days, weeks, or months of blaming are never as satisfying or as productive as the minutes required to decide that you are the only one who can live your life and improve your health — and therefore clearly and confidently assume full responsibility for it.

Taking responsibility for your health by deciding to shape a wellness lifestyle is a liberating act. It can be a source of immense satisfaction to realize that your own beliefs, attitudes, and actions have more to do with your level of well-being than do the hundreds of millions spent on health insurance, hospitals, doctors, drugs, and all the rest.

The Annual Report from the University of Wisconsin–Stevens Point Health Service and Lifestyle Improvement

Program in 1980 contained a graph, reproduced below, showing the factors that contribute most to the quality and enjoyment of life. Quoting from the Report:

> While it is true that doctors and hospitals have a significant role to play in the quality of our lives, this graph clearly indicates that it is individuals, through the choices that they make each day, that contribute the greatest percentage toward maximizing the quality of life and health. We all know that our behaviors can improve our chances for leading a long and useful life. Collectively, all of our behaviors can be described as our lifestyle.*

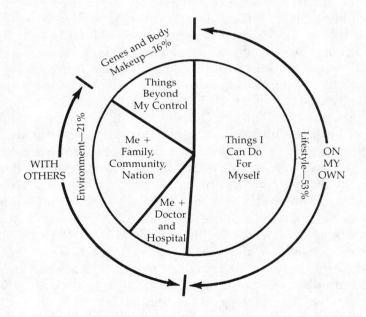

*"In Pursuit of Wellness," Annual Report FY 80 (University Health Service & Lifestyle Improvement Program, 1980), p. 677.

Unfortunately, health educators have made very little effort to promote the joys and satisfactions that go with self-responsibility. No wonder they have been called "warriors against pleasure." (I'm reminded of H.L. Mencken, the great "puritan smiter," who said these forefathers of health educators were possessed with a haunting fear that someone, somewhere, may be happy.) I'm partially exaggerating, as usual; a few health educators *have* emphasized the central role of self-responsibility and the benefits that it enables. But not many.

There are many ways to describe self-responsibility. In *High Level Wellness,* I called it the philosopher's stone, the mariner's compass, and the ring of power to a wellness lifestyle. However expressed, this *is* the keystone to realizing your best potentials; *the* greatest health problem today is the forfeiture of health to someone or something else.

John Knowles, late president of the Rockefeller Foundation and a prominent public policy-shaping physician, discussed self-responsibility at length in his writings. Knowles argued that the costs of failed personal responsibility are assumed by the public, that a quest for "rights" has distracted most from acknowledging accountability, and that the improvement of health levels will only come when personal responsibility for health is widely acknowledged. Excerpts from his essay should be insightful:

The idea of individual responsibility has been submerged to individual rights — rights, or demands, to be guaranteed by government and delivered by public and private institutions. The cost of sloth, gluttony, alcoholic intemperance, reckless driving, sexual frenzy, and smoking is now a national, and not an individual, responsibility. This is justified as individual freedom — but one man's freedom in health is another man's shackle in taxes and insurance premiums. I believe the idea of a "right" to health should be replaced by the idea of an individual moral obligation to preserve one's own health — a public duty if you will. The individual then has the "right" to expect help with information, accessible services of good quality, and minimal barriers . . .

Nader's Raiders have yet to allow that the next major advances in the health of the American people will come from the assumption of individual responsibility for one's own health and a necessary change in habits for the majority of Americans . . . . The barriers to the assumption of individual responsibility for one's own health are lack of knowledge . . .lack of sufficient interest in, and knowledge about, what is preventable and the "cost-to-benefit" ratios of nationwide health programs, and a culture which has progressively eroded the idea of individual responsibility while stressing individual rights, the responsibility of society-at-large, and the steady growth of production and consumption ("We have met the enemy and it is us!").*

Dr. John Travis, founder of the Wellness Resource Center and author of the *Wellness Workbook,* discusses self-responsibility in relation "to your points of view" toward any given event. Travis notes that many points of view are possible with regard to any circumstance (e.g., seeing your parked car demolished by a drunken driver). An emotion is behind each viewpoint. The composite of our viewpoints is our "act" (e.g., "nice guy act," "tough bastard act," etc.), and current acts are usually based on what "worked" in childhood. Travis suggests taking responsibility for updating our acts in accord with our higher selves and choosing viewpoints that lead to optimal health. Quoting Travis:

---

*John H. Knowles, "The Responsibility of the Individual," in *Doing Better and Feeling Worse: Health in the United States. Daedalus, Journal of the American Academy of Arts and Sciences,* Winter, 1977, pp. 5-60.

Taking full responsibility for your life and your health can only come when you step back from your attachment to your viewpoints and your acts, and realize that you chose them. Since you chose them, you can decide to choose different ones any time you find that the current ones are not working. Gradually you can create for yourself a world view which is in harmony with yourself and your environment.*

Pelletier sees self-responsibility as one essential characteristic of those who choose to rise above the "pathologies of normalcy":

The new sense of personal responsibility extends into the realization that one can exercise choice regarding whether to be subjected to the brutalization of the evening news, the monstrous routine of an occupation which has ceased to be anything other than monetarily rewarding, or the unduly restrictive censure of a partner or peer group.†

The increasing popularity of high-level wellness has led to many expressions and interpretations of self-responsibility. I think the following excerpt from the annual report of a New Jersey foundation that supports two innovative wellness programs is worth citing in this context:

Recently, attention has been given to the idea that in certain key ways the citizen bears first responsibility for his own health. This applies for all citizens, whether they reside in suburbia or the ghetto. An irony of American life is that even the poor suffer primarily from outlooks and indulgences spawned

---

*John W. Travis, *Wellness Workbook* (Mill Valley, CA: Wellness Resource Center, 1977), p. 82.
†Kenneth R. Pelletier, *Mind As Healer, Mind As Slayer* (New York: Delta, 1977), p. 303.

by affluence. Advances in transportation reduce the exercise which comes from walking. Television fosters sedentary routines. A plethora of fast cars kills more of us than most of the dread diseases kill in any emerging nation.

It is probably true that more Americans suffer from abdicated responsibility than from denied rights. And it is with that in mind that Victoria [Foundation, Inc.] is starting to promote self-responsibility for maintaining Wellness, in the belief that it is even more important than the availability of sophisticated medical care.

Wellness is being promoted with the realization that certain life-damaging habits are difficult to break and that wholesome lifestyles are not necessarily alluring, especially when force-fed. It is believed, however, that properly presented, fundamental components of preventive medicine and health education can be inculcated in the minds and habits of the young. Run-away costs of traditional health services offer an economic incentive for Wellness in addition to its intrinsic value.*

All of this is a way of saying that you are the source of what you are, what you do, and what you have. This point of view extends to include responsibility for most of what is done to you.

Responsibility is not the same as fault, blame or guilt. These are judgments and evaluations of good and bad, right and wrong, or better and worse. They get in the way of a simple acknowledgment that you are the root of your own experience.

Wellness can also be defined in the context of how you choose to experience yourself, as explained by physician

---

*Victoria Foundation Inc., 1978 Annual Report, Montclair, New Jersey, p. 11.

Ron Pion:

You are in charge of your state of being. You have learned to be exactly the way you are and you have the remarkable human capability to learn to be another way. Choosing the ways of thinking, feeling and doing which contribute to your health pleasures rather than your health problems is the nitty gritty of being *well*.*

WHAT SELF-RESPONSIBILITY MEANS

Self-responsibility means that you see yourself as the sovereign, king/queen, commander-in-chief, President for Life, Conqueror of the British Empire, Ayatollah, or whatever solemn (or ridiculous) title you can imagine to represent that you see yourself as the primo agent for your well-being. The implications of taking this position are nearly limitless, but the prerequisites for "black belt" accountability status can be identified. Let's look at a number of characteristics of advanced responsibility.

· **A conscious commitment to your own well-being.** In the famous *Screwtape Letters*, C.S. Lewis (with tongue in cheek) has the devil admonish his nephew to forego efforts of a dramatic and sudden nature to lure souls into hell. Far more effective, suggests the devil, are the little temptations and dissolutions spread over the long haul of the years. Notes the devil:

The surest and safest road to hell is the gradual one, soft under foot, without sudden turnings, without signposts, without milestones.

---

*Ronald J. Pion, *A Prescription for Wellness*. For copies of this ten-page booklet, write for it by name at Suite 518, 8920 Wilshire Blvd., Beverly Hills, CA 90211.

In other words, people can slide, over time, into low-level worseness. In Lewis's story, the "slide" is eternal perdition (Hades); for our purposes, it involves dissolution (obesity, sedentary and stress-filled lives, empty jobs, unhappy relationships, etc.). Unless, of course, a conscious, aware decision is made to pursue the heights. When you acknowledge and act upon self-responsibility for your own health, you arrest the slow and inexorable drift into mediocre lifestyles. In addition, taking responsibility keeps you from going all to hell — on Earth or elsewhere.

· **The avoidance of high-risk behaviors.** It is difficult to convince yourself, let alone others, that you are serious about wellness if you model self-destructive habits such as smoking, the misuse of alcohol, or other forms of self-abuse. You no doubt are aware of all the ugly conditions that are caused by smoking (ranging from diseases to hair on the palms to bad breath), but there is another drawback that seldom is talked about. It is the "I'm a loser syndrome" — the bizarre desire of smokers to display to their friends and others the fact that they are emotionally off-center, angry with themselves, and hell-bent on diminishing their fading hopes for approaching physical and other potentials. Why put yourself in the back of the bus/airplane? Why crowd in with the greasers, hoodlums, and assorted riff-raff? There is a reason for the inverse relationship between the presence of high-risk behaviors and the acceptance and pursuit of personal responsibility — it is that the presence of one blocks out the other. For you and anyone else interested in wellness, it should be no contest in a choice between the two.

· **An understanding of the limits of medicine.** As emphasized in Day Three, studies have repeatedly shown that of the four health determinants (lifestyle, environment, heredity, and health care), health care is the least important. The death-rate decline over the past century is not a condition of medical advances; in fact, the gains in life expectancy are attributed primarily to environmental advances which have provided controls over infectious diseases. Health is best where doctors are fewest, suggests Vickery*, whose first medical myth is that health depends most on medical care. There is little evidence to support the effectiveness of as much as 90 percent of the medical procedures on which Americans spend vast sums of money, and for which they literally risk life and limb. A 1978 study by the Office of Technology Assessment, an agency of the Congress, found that medical procedures for tonsillectomy, mastectomy, appendectomy, hysterectomy, and four different coronary surgeries are without proven worth.† Add to that Vickery's claim that there is no evidence of effectiveness for annual physical examinations, multiphasic screening, blood tests for diabetes, X-rays for lung cancer, and blood tests for anemia, gout, arthritis, and thyroid disease, and you start to get the picture. There are occasions when medical care is useful (injuries, breast exams, blood pressure checks, Pap smears, and so forth), but it is both dangerous and expensive to delegate responsibility for your health to practitioners of the treatment arts.

· **A realization, introduced on Day One, that health is vastly more than not being sick.** In order to assume the role of prime mover in designing and living a wellness lifestyle, you have to be clear about the benefits of personal responsibility. Knowing that there are "worlds to conquer," or at least superb horizons of physical excellence to achieve through exercise and other efforts, provides the source motivation to strengthen the self-responsibility ethic.

· **An ability to practice self-care and use the medical sys-**

---

*Donald M. Vickery, *Lifeplan for Your Health* (New York: Addison-Wesley, 1978), p. 7.
†"Medical Practices Called Unproven," *The Nation's Health,* American Public Health Association, November, 1978, p. 12.

tem effectively. If you break your leg, you want qualified medical treatment. This is an example of an easy decision; some issues are not so evident. What about X-rays, the length of stay in hospitals, the number of tests that seem appropriate for diagnostic (versus defensive medicine) purposes, family medical records, and similar matters? Do you have a sense for what is enough as against what is too much? Do you know where to obtain independent opinions on these kind of issues? Most important, are you willing and interested in investing the modest time and energy required to get this and other self-care information? If so, credit yourself with a strong sense of responsibility in relation to the appropriate use of the medical system. Your chances of suffering iatrogenesis (doctor-caused illness), needless testing expenses and hazards, and disproportionate costs are much lower than average.*

· **Your wisdom in being able to dispense with or at least be conscious of the right/wrong game.** Perhaps your parents, friends, and/or associates have modeled "blaming" patterns to the extent that you do likewise. If so, consider the advantages of discarding such tendencies. An alternative that is easier to live with is to look upon events or actions by others as just the way things or people are; that it or they need to be as they are at that point in time; and that emotional pain or "hurt" about it will not change things, or profit you in any conceivable fashion. With this outlook you are free of futile judgments about how unfair life is or how wrong other persons are. You are free of the terrible burden of having to be right all the time. You become more tolerant of others and accepting of yourself. You can, in other words, be responsible without being in control of all the variables.

---

*An excellent source of such information is the quarterly magazine *Medical Self Care*, $15 per year, from P.O. Box 717, Inverness, CA 94937.

· **Your success in cultivating skills in the area of responsible sex.** Assuming you are as interested in the subject as I am, it is in your interest as well as that of your current or future partner to appreciate the rewards of considerate sex. There are only a few requirements for responsible human sexuality, all of which involve being aware of your needs and those of your partner! (When you do not involve others, things are much simpler, if less challenging.) It is, in my opinion, poor form not to talk about whatever considerations are important to you or potentially so to your partner or partners. For example, birth control, VD, and confidentiality are among the issues that ought to be discussed "out front." "Is there anything I should know?" "Are you protected?" "Will anyone be hurt by our enjoyment?" I realize these are not lines of classic high romance; they are nowhere to be found in any of Shakespeare's plays, and Rudolph Valentino would have been a wallflower if these were the best he came up with. But they are illustrative of considerate efforts to prevent upsets. Assume responsibility and you enhance the sexual experience for all involved. Find your own words to engage in the kind of awareness foreplay that will benefit everybody — responsible people make better lovers.

· **The amount of effort you put into developing an internal locus of control.** Psychologists, social researchers, health educators, and others* have developed scales that measure the degree to which you perceive your health to be a condition of your own actions or a matter of luck, fate, chance, or powerful others (e.g., doctors). The kinds of questions asked are as follows: the rating scale ranges from strong disagreement (one point) through strong agreement (six points). Mark your points to the right of each question.

---

*See B.S. Wallston, et al., "Development and Validation of the Health Locus of Control Scale," *Journal of Consult Clinical Psychology* 44 (1976): pp. 580-85.

1. When I become ill, it's a matter of fate.

2. I can pretty much stay healthy by taking good care of myself.

3. Even when I take care of myself, it's easy to get sick.

4. When I stay healthy, I'm just plain lucky.

5. My physical well-being depends on how well I take care of myself.

6. When I am sick, I just have to let nature run its course.

7. Whatever goes wrong with my health is my own fault.

8. It seems that my health is greatly influenced by accidental happenings.

9. I am directly responsible for my health.

10. Often I feel that no matter what I do, if I am going to get sick, I will get sick.

11. If I become sick, I have the power to make myself well again.

You are big on personal responsibility if you scored a 5 or 6 on questions 2, 5, 6, 9, and 11.

A few other characteristics of self-responsibility include the extent to which one is sanguine about the motives of others, the extent of belief in the goodness of human nature, faith in first impressions, belief in the predictability of human nature, and the extent to which one feels rewarded in life by one's own actions. Just to consider these perspectives can be a helpful consciousness raiser. Think of where you stand on these matters: do what you can to move farther toward the self-reliant, personal-accountability side of the scale.

· **Your willingness to allow others to find their own paths.**

There are important differences between helping others when asked and getting in their way when your counsel is neither invited nor desired. People must be open and willing to listen before they will be influenced by suggestions or advice. Try to talk a person into joining you for a 14-Day wellness lifestyle experiment if that person is not ready for it, and he/she might act as if he/she just underwent a charisma bypass.

I know this from personal experience. Who do you think shows up for my lectures on wellness? I'll tell you: the true believers, the paragons of wellness, the savants of superhealth, the "choir" of the already-converted-to-optimal-health — in short, the healthiest people in town. They do not "need" to hear me run on about wellness — they already know it is terrific. They turn out because they want to reinforce their current practices and hear someone lionize the virtues of their current lifestyles. Those who could benefit the most from hearing a pitch for optimal pathways to health enrichment seldom appear. They are too busy practicing middle-level mediocrity, or worse.

I was booked by mistake a while ago as the keynote speaker for a convention of inebriated, chain-smoking Valium salesmen. (They expected Rodney Dangerfield. He ended up at the National Jogging Association.) You think the pill pushers wanted to hear about wellness?

The moral is: Do not be the Carrie Nation of wellness. Be sensitive to where your friends and associates are on the Worseness/Wellness Continuum. Be especially considerate of the extent to which the other person is or is not in a psychological place to hear about wellness. Unsolicited advice does not promote adoption of self-responsibility; in fact, such advice-giving has been termed "rescuing." In transactional analysis, rescuing is considered neither effective nor appreciated, and often leads to mutual feelings of being victimized. Rescuers, it seems, often neglect their own needs, become "stroke" or acknowledgment-de-

prived, and are thereby unlikely to meet their own requirements in an effective way. So, step back and give people
room. When they are on the pathway or open to hearing
about moving in that direction, you will know. Take responsibility for your own situation and get your own act
organized before you rescue the natives, heathens, and
other lost souls. Keep in mind the difference between helping and rescuing.

· **Your capacity to understand and accept what you can —
and cannot — affect.** Most people *underestimate* their power
and creativity. While none of us can fly, trade parents, or
achieve immortality, there remain a lot of options! With a
plan, a strong will, a commitment to goals, patience, and a
bit of luck, you can surprise yourself and amaze your
friends. There is just one important rule in taking responsibility for this aspect of health and well-being: *focus your
energies on realistic expectations and outcomes.* Build a record of
small neighborhood successes before taking on the
Everests of the world. The little accomplishments will
strengthen your confidence and self-esteem. Try not to get
grim and serious about a goal — you can do just as well with
a sense of humor and perspective.

· **Your readiness to interpret setbacks as hidden opportunities.** Things will not always go well. Even if your parents, peers, and circumstances gave you an enormous head
start, via good genetics, habits, and opportunities, you will
almost surely have some illness days, even if you practice
wellness all out. For instance, if you are active in sports,
you may get injured on occasion. All this is part of the larger
game — when it happens, try not to be much upset about it.
It does you no good to be demoralized or angry. The amazing thing about "setbacks" is that you can use them to make
advances! Suppose you are looking ahead to a hot date and,
the day before the great event, crack your big toe practicing
karate. No problem, if you interpret the situation in a crea-

tive manner. Maybe you can't boogie at the hop, but you can get better acquainted in other ways. In more serious cases involving the loss of people you love, missed opportunities, rejections, and so forth, it is your viewpoint that makes all the difference. If your viewpoint will allow it, you can find meaning and new direction in each setback. It is natural, and even functional at times, to be hurt, sad, grieved, and so forth — for a spell, but move on as soon as possible.

Did you know there were over 100 participants in the Boston, Honolulu, and New York marathons who belonged to the "Broken Heart Club," a group composed exclusively of men and women who have suffered heart attacks. Few if any thought, before the death of a piece of their heart, that they would one day run 26-plus miles. However, a dreadful crisis (heart attack) provided the "opportunity" to reassess a lifestyle, make a dramatic change in exercise and other habit patterns, and pursue optimal health rather than minimal survival.

You do not have to experience such risky depths to know that any setback has within it the potentials for growth — in fact, for transformation. If things look really grim, remember: "There are no unsolvable problems; there are only undiscovered solutions."

· **Your success in overcoming temptations to rely on gurus.** I have nothing against gurus. Some of them may be very fine folks — a few no doubt operate at an elevated level of consciousness and are probably highly evolved spiritual beings. But the term has been used in recent years to describe cult leaders who tend to attract fervent devotees. Followers tend to practice unquestioning obedience to the master and religious adoption of his sacrosanct approaches. There can be no guru or gurus in *this* program because there cannot, by definition, be uncritical followers in wellness. This is a lifestyle that embodies personal reliance and unique pathways. You find your own ways to integrate what works for you in each of the wellness dimensions, in accord with your extraordinary individuality in background, values, preferences, history, and needs. The temptation in every area of human endeavor is to find a leader and emulate him/her. In wellness, this will not work, as it contradicts self-responsibility, the foundation of the wellness ethic. Furthermore, a wellness lifestyle is simply too all-encompassing to make guru watching feasible; your interests in fitness, stress awareness and management, and nutrition are unique. No guru could have much success in trying to convince you to follow a single way. The idea of anyone being able to lead you about in a movement that starts with self-responsibility is, in fact, contradictory. Remember, you are the guru for your own well-being. Consider what experts, real and self-appointed, have to say, evaluate what might work for you, and make your own choices!

· **Your commitment to eradicating "no-win" beliefs.** Everyone is exposed to certain mythologies as he/she grows up, and some take them too seriously. When this happens, impossible standards, rules, and expectations are created at an unconscious level. Thus, traps are set and *you* get caught in them — every day.

Here are a few such traps to recognize and dismantle, by deciding that you are not going to put yourself in such no-win positions any longer:

- · Things should always go well.
- · Life should be fair — always.
- · Justice must be done.
- · Right will prevail.
- · Nobody will be selfish.
- · You must understand the past (e.g., why your mother treated you as she did) to cope in the present.
- · Somewhere out there is your perfect mate.

- If it is good for you, it has to hurt.
- I cannot like myself if others disapprove.
- More money, a better job, a new lover, etc., will make me happy (i.e., "Things go better with Coke").

You get the idea. There is just enough "reasonableness" in all these positions to make them seductive, attractive, and believable, which will in turn guarantee constant upset, trauma, ingrown toenails, and a serious persecution complex. There are countless other statements like the above that encourage little voices in your head to question your judgments and otherwise try to make you feel guilty or outraged, disappointed or resigned. Don't be fooled. There will be times when you are not perfect! You will make a few mistakes, setbacks will occur, illness will develop, and so on. Life is *not* fair all the time. Injustice sometimes wins out.

The wellness measures are: What attitudes serve you, are consistent with your standards, and contribute to or at least do not harm others? Life is challenging enough without having to deal with self-defeating expectations. Take responsibility for acknowledging the lurking presence of such no-win beliefs, and excuse them from your life.

Well, my responsible friend, I realize this Day's reading got a bit lengthy, but there is no more critical variable affecting your commitment to a wellness lifestyle than your enthusiasm for "hoarding" the maximum amount of accountability. As Mae West might put it: "You can't get too much of a good thing — like responsibility for your own health and destiny." So glory in it. The more you "exaggerate" your role in your own life events, the larger that role will become and the better your realizations will be. And, pretty soon, you will understand that self-responsibility cannot *be* exaggerated — it is always as great as you make it.

You worked for this one — give yourself a bold, self-responsible check for Day Six.

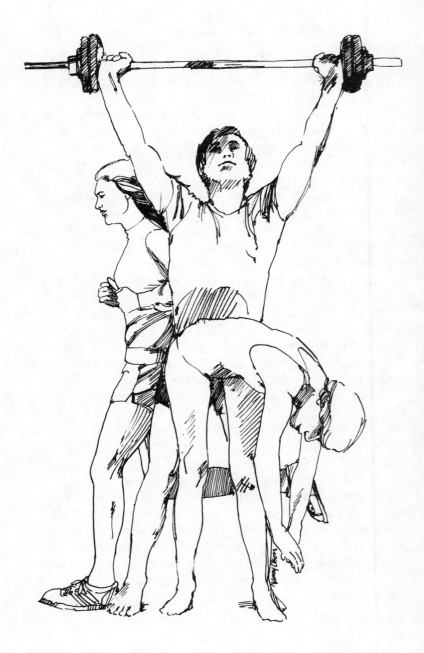

Day Seven

Consider The Enormous Payoffs Of Physical Fitness And The Adequacy Requirements Of Any Exercise

Purpose: By the completion of this Day, you should be informed about and committed to physical fitness as a prerequisite element of a wellness lifestyle, and aware of frequency, intensity, and duration as *the* measures of exercise adequacy.

Here is what to expect of Day Seven in a sentence or two. A summary of good reasons to exercise (even if you now hate exercise) that revolve around nasty conditions which you avoid. This is called a negative rationale, but it is still a good one. A summary of other good reasons for exercise that entails positive satisfactions which reinforce and reward physical excellence. The latter are considered the best reasons. When the Day is complete, you will be more interested in these payoffs, knowledgeable about the types of exercise needed and other requirements essential for optimal fitness routines. Enjoy the Day.

THE PAYOFFS — POSITIVE AND OTHERWISE

Until recently in human history, you had to be fit to survive. If you could not flee, fight, hunt, swim, and otherwise move about in short time spans under your own power, you would be left for the buzzards. Guess what? The forms have changed (there's a buzzard shortage), but the outcome is the same. If you are unfit, less opportunities and satisfactions will come your way, and more people will leave you behind. To be fit is to be able to play life's game with all the best equipment and preparation under optimal conditions. To be in poor shape is to handicap yourself unnecessarily, making life so much more difficult than necessary.

There is no shortage of books, articles, tapes, and posters (not to mention proselytizing fitness buffs) which describe in detail all the dreadful diseases and infirmities that await the unfit. Wellness is a positive approach, so I'll spare you the long lists of awful problems that face the sedentary person, ranging from back pains to hypertension, obesity, premature aging, cardiovascular disasters, and furniture disease.*

There are just two basic reasons why you should put a lot of energy into this wellness dimension. One of these reasons is a rationale that is essentially negative, that is, seeks to avoid something; the other is positive. The latter, naturally, is best; so I will summarize the negative first and get it out of the way. It concerns the consequences of degeneration: if you do not exercise, *everything* that you want to stay up goes down. Worse, what you want to keep down goes up — and stays that way! Let me explain. What goes down is cardiovascular capacity, lean body mass, muscle strength and endurance, flexibility, respiratory efficiency (including rate, capacity, residual volume, musculature, and resistance to air flow), and self-satisfaction with your own body image. What goes up leads to "Disaster City":

---

* An embarrassing condition wherein your chest drops into your drawers.

increased spread of the waist, hips, and butt; greater body weight (i.e., obesity — and beyond); more body fat relative to lean muscle tissue; higher blood pressure; elevated cholesterol and triglycerides; and raised heart rates. What a bummer!

Look at it another way. Fit employees are more effective. Here is why. When you are fit, you dramatically slow the decline of your body's functional capacity as you age. Without a fitness routine, your heart and lungs will perform less efficiently, bones become fragile, joints stiffen, muscle strength declines, and you absorb less oxygen during exertion. All this, of course, affects both physical and mental work ability, not to mention one's opportunities for total living. If the heart cannot get enough blood to the working muscles and tissues, you will fade before your time. It is estimated that sedentary individuals deteriorate 40 percent between the ages of 35 and 70. After that (more often, sometime during this decline), the immune systems break down, tumors appear, and the downward course accelerates to its inevitable conclusion — decades prematurely. What a loss.

These are negative aspects that warn of the consequences of *not* exercising. People have almost always lined up to stay away when health educators start preaching about the hazards of this or that. Young people, for example, are avidly uninterested in avoiding illness, but very much interested in experiencing advanced health — and fitness deserves to be discussed in this positive context.

Continuing the up/down analogy, let's emphasize the values and gains that derive from *doing* regular exercise — the second rationale for embracing this wellness dimension. Let us try to forget all the ghastly things that occur if fitness is slighted or ignored. These issues involve vitalization achievement, not degeneration avoidance. Investigators who study "hard core" fitness buffs usually note the presence of high levels of spontaneity, creativity, playfulness, and self-esteem. By being fit, you have an added reserve of energy *after* you have completed all the basic things you have to do to get by (at school, work, and so forth). You have added zest for the optional things in life that make living enjoyable and fulfilling, and that enable excellence in things that matter most.

The Canadian government has done a lot to promote fitness. After declaring that the average twenty-seven-year-old Canadian had the fitness level of a sixty-two-year-old Swede (which had to hurt national pride), the Ministry of Health and Welfare went on to identify varied fitness programs in half their proposed health promotion strategies. The Canadian position supports the wellness notion that the true value of fitness goes far beyond survival and illness avoidance to the celebration of human possibilities and an adaptation to a fuller existence. In recent years, the Canadian Ministry of Culture and Recreation (Ontario) has sponsored a project known as Fitness Ontario. This organization conducts a wide range of fitness educational services and opportunities, and publishes a variety of guides and booklets. Research in Canada and the U.S. shows that high levels of total-body conditioning produce the following states: strengthened heart/lungs and related cardiovascular and pulmonary functions, lowered blood pressure, improved oxygenation and circulation of nutrients to body tissues, increased metabolic rates, and better muscle tone. When sedentary people take up and stay with well-designed fitness programs, they experience (in addition to the above gains) such benefits as improved digestion and elimination, lower cholesterol and triglycerides, more high-density lipoproteins (HDLs), formation of new collateral blood vessels and capillaries, greater immunity to illness, and lower resting and recovery heart rates.*

Many investigators of the fitness phenomenon believe the psychological benefits are even better than the physical

---

*Donald B. Ardell, "The Physical Disciplines and Health," *Health for the Whole Person: The Complete Guide to Holistic Medicine,* ed. Arthur C. Hastings et al. Boulder, CO (Westview Press, 1980), pp. 191-208.

gains. These payoffs include, but are not limited to, the following: feeling and looking better, experiencing more energy and productivity, increased self-confidence and personal esteem, and higher levels of endurance and resistance to illness. If that is not enough, consider the reports of better body image and weight loss, slower aging processes, enhancement of sexuality, improved emotional balance, more graceful and coordinated movements, greater personal power, and raised overall effectiveness.

Given all this, it is no wonder that organized medicine is beginning to recognize that physical activity is not an option but an integral part of the healthy life. As noted in a prestigious medical journal, physical inactivity is seen as "far more detrimental to health than any hazards of strenuous exertion.... Anyone should submit to a thorough medical checkup before deciding not to exercise."* Today, it is the inactive person who is advised to get the stress test, to see how long he/she might survive the rigors of a sedentary lifestyle. What a turnaround in thinking from just a few years ago.

This leads to the presence today of a curious paradox. On the one hand, more people than ever before are engaged in strenuous physical activities (e.g., 50,000 Americans have run at least one marathon, according to the President's Council on Physical Fitness and Sports). On the other, more than 70 percent of the population does not exercise adequately or often enough, according to the same source. What is going on? What accounts for this situation where some get more than enough but most get too little? Surely, there is a complex set of factors at work, but three seem predominant: excessive attention to negative messages ("use it or lose it"), insufficient focus on positive payoffs, and inadequate understanding of how much of what kind of exercise is (better than) adequate.

---

*Ralph S. Paffenbarger and Robert T. Hyde, "Exercise As Protection Against Heart Disease," *The New England Journal of Medicine* (May, 1980), pp. 1026-27.

The first two have been given enough attention to this point. You surely realize that there are unpleasant consequences of being a slothful, lazy bum, but that the greatest loss would be missed satisfactions, and the joys of a life of vigor and activity.

That took several pages to communicate. Enough — you probably agreed with all this to begin with. It is time to define the specific types of exercise and the measures of adequacy to insure that, whatever you do, you both avoid the negative and enjoy the positive outcomes.

MEASURES OF ADEQUACY FOR PHYSICAL FITNESS

Please recognize that there are no established standards of physical excellence; there are only varied opinions about minimal adequacy. Wellness goes far beyond adequacy, but this is a useful place to start.

Once underway, you should plan to leave normalcy, adequacy, and minimal standards in your wake. Depending on the level of attention you give to nutrition and all the other variables, plus innate capabilities, the energy you will want to invest in physical fitness will be unique to your situation. What will represent superior performance and high-level capacity for you cannot be established or even estimated without elaborate physiologic testing. (This may or may not be of interest to you. It is not the focus of this Day's discussion.)

This commentary deals with baseline concepts with which you can assess your exercise routines. Using these measures, you can avoid or at least greatly reduce your exposure to premature infirmities (i.e., negative consequences of inadequate exercise) and enhance your prospects for positive returns.

First, realize that there are three different kinds of exercise: endurance (or aerobic exercise), strength building, and flexibility. All three are important and all should be accomplished on a regular basis.

Of the three, endurance/aerobic, or what is basically cardiorespiratory training deserves, demands, and almost always involves the largest amount of attention. This is the steady, rhythmic activity that does not lead to oxygen debt. It utilizes and strengthens your general musculature, develops more efficient lungs, a more powerful heart, and a better vascular system. Examples of endurance exercise activities include walking, jogging, cross-country skiing, swimming, biking, and rope jumping. Any activity done at a steady pace over an extended period of time that requires elevated heart rates qualifies as endurance training.

Some of these activities may seem intimidating if you have not engaged in a regular fitness routine for some time. But don't worry: walking is available and completely satisfactory if you are not in the best of shape. Just take off on a walk from your house for ten or fifteen minutes, and turn around and return. Make a routine of this; convert the walk into a ritual part of your day. You will derive all the benefits noted above. Save the hike up Mt. Everest for later.

A second exercise type is strength building. It involves muscle power (force) and endurance. It is the ability of a muscle group to persist in a given activity in which localized fatigue rather than general exhaustion is the limiting factor. It includes dynamic (repetitions) and static (holding or pausing during a weight lift) muscle contractions. Examples include chin-ups, push-ups, certain calisthenics, Nautilus training, pumping iron, and the like.

Flexibility is the third kind of exercise. It entails a range of movement activities in the structure of joints and the soft tissue around the joints. It occurs, for instance, during warm-up/warm-down stretching routines. It is an important activity for preventing lower-back pains, avoiding muscle and joint injuries, and in improving performance by delaying the onset of muscle fatigue. Two areas of principle concern when developing increased flexibility are the lower-back and hamstring muscles. Yoga is one example of an excellent flexibility form.

The three established standards of adequacy pertain primarily to the major type of exercise, namely, endurance or aerobic (cardiovascular) training. The three standards are intensity, frequency, and duration.

Intensity is a measure of how hard or vigorous the activity is for any given individual. Obviously, there are enormous differences among humans in terms of the intensity involved in, say, running ten miles. Craig Virgin could cover this distance in hiking boots and toga in less than 50 minutes; most Americans cannot safely run ten miles. For Craig, such a jog might be mildly intensive (he would breathe hard and sweat); for most everyone else (including me), running (or attempting to run) at such a pace for a tenth of this distance would be hazardously intensive! The same differences apply to biking, swimming, or anything — our capacities vary. Yet, while everyone has his or her limits which cannot be generalized at the high end (the heights of potentials), the minimals are known to a reasonably accurate degree. Another way to express this issue of a minimal exercise standard of intensity is to ask: How hard is hard enough? What is required in order to derive substantial benefit from endurance or aerobic exercise? Remembering that the question is only related to what in a wellness context is viewed as a negative but still useful motive (i.e., disease avoidance), the answer is (you guess):

A. 60% of your cardiovascular work capacity if you are in poor shape;
B. 70% of your cardiovascular work capacity if you are in fair/good shape;
C. 70-85% of your cardiovascular work capacity if you are in great shape;
D. Any rate up to the point where you can still converse, stay out of oxygen debt (which occurs when the exercising muscles require more oxygen than the cardiovascular system can deliver), and not experience obvious signs of overexertion (such as tight-

ness or pain in the chest, severe breathlessness, lightheadedness, dizziness, loss of muscle control and nausea, imminent unconsciousness, or sudden death);

E. All of the above are discussed as guides in the literature on training for fitness.

The correct choice, of course, is "E."

The standard of intensity is most often linked with heart rate. Here are two heartbeat-monitoring intensity charts published by Fitness Ontario; chart A is for beginners, chart B is not. (The last column on the right refers to the ten-second count used to determine your exercise heart rate.)*

CHART A

Age	Exercise Heart Rate Lower Limit Upper Limit	No. of Beats in 10 Seconds
20-30	approx. 110 to 150 beats/min.	approx. 18 to 25
31-40	approx. 110 to 138 beats/min.	approx. 18 to 23
41-50	approx. 96 to 126 beats/min.	approx. 16 to 21
51-60	approx. 90 to 114 beats/min.	approx. 15 to 19

CHART B

Age	Exercise Heart Rate Lower Limit Upper Limit	No. of Beats in 10 Seconds
20-30	approx. 144 to 174 beats/min.	approx. 24 to 29
31-40	approx. 132 to 162 beats/min.	approx. 22 to 27
41-50	approx. 120 to 150 beats/min.	approx. 20 to 25
51-60	approx. 108 to 138 beats/min.	approx. 18 to 23

A Guide to Personal Fitness (Fitness Ontario, no date), p. 8.

The second established standard of adequacy is frequency. "How often must one exercise to develop an immunity of sorts against heart disease or some other infirmity?" is the way the frequency issue is usually addressed. The answers vary. Many try not to scare potential exercisers off. They might cross their fingers and say, "Three to five times per week." The President's Council urges "five exercise sessions per week, at least." Others, such as Ralph Paffenbarger, M.D., of Stanford University, claim that data from about 17,000 Harvard alumni suggest that at least four hours per week (enough to burn 2,000 or more calories through exercise) is the minimal figure. The AMA, and nearly all wellness centers, encourage daily exercise.

The third standard of exercise adequacy is duration, or how long? The President's Council* states 20 minutes per exercise session, in the beginning, working up to 45 minutes as conditioning improves.

To summarize, intensity/frequency/duration measures are useful for insuring that you derive the "training effect" from whatever endurance program you choose. Opinions vary, but the widest consensus is for exercise at about 70 percent of maximum intensity done five times per week for approximately 45 minutes. If your aerobic exercise meets these standards, and you supplement such activity with flexibility and strength-building efforts, you are doing very well.

There are four general principles you should know that affect conditioning. These are *specificity, overload, adaptation,* and *progression.* An appreciation of these concepts will be of great use to you as you advance from exercise levels that meet the minimum standards of adequacy to that level consistent with (and deserving of) your capabilities.

The results or advances in terms of physical fitness from any activity — whether primarily endurance, strength-

---

*For interesting free information, including booklets and an award program, write the President's Council on Physical Fitness and Sports, Washington, D.C. 20201.

building, or flexibility — are specific to the type of that activity. Exercise that is intense will develop strength and power; efforts of long duration build endurance or cardiorespiratory fitness. In addition, the effects of exercise are specific to the particular body functions or muscle groups which a given activity develops. If you run ten miles a day for six months and one afternoon join in a vigorous game of touch football on the beach, you will be extremely sore the next day. The "football muscles" were on vacation during all the months of running; the reverse would also hold. The *specificity* principle is a good reason for participating in a variety of fitness activities, as well as obtaining a balance of exercise in the three basic types of conditioning.

The second general principle affecting conditioning is that of *overload*. In order to improve any muscle group or function, it is necessary to place that group or perform that function under a greater than normal workload. By doing so, the function gradually adapts to the greater workload. The degree of improvement is directly proportional to the degree of the overload in a unit of time. That is, to overload successfully, the physical stress of increased exercise must be greater in intensity or duration than the demands normally placed on the organism.

Cardiovascular conditioning is a case of overloading the heart muscle. When taxed close to the maximum (i.e., 70%), it grows stronger, larger, and more efficient. Exercises such as long-distance running, cycling, and cross-country skiing, for instance, entail sufficient duration and intensity workloads to provide these conditioning advances.

Adaptation is the third principle with which you should be familiar. It refers to the physiological (and psychological) adjustments by the organism to the stresses encountered in the process of overload. Your present state of fitness or the shape you are in is the result of a complex series of adaptations your body has made over the years to the exercise requirements you placed upon it. The body is an amazing vehicle for transporting you through life. It will adapt just as surely to a low-level-worseness state of physical ruin as to a wellness lifestyle of high performance. Put another way, think of your body as the raw material for a sluggish, broken-down heap or a rocketlike marvel of efficiency. If your body were an automobile, which of the following would it most resemble?

A. A used sedan just retired from the fleet at Yellow Cab Co.
B. A late-model 4-door Mercedes diesel.
C. A no-frills cutdown 1500-pound chassis powered by a 560-horsepower Cosworth turbocharged V-8.

The better question might be: What type of machine (body capability) do you want to possess a year from now? The path to advanced functioning is along the way of adaptation over time — at a pace that works for you. You have a unique potential that spans an even greater range than indicated by this little auto analogy. By changing your expectations and attendant activities, you can adapt for physical excellence.

Before taking off in rapid pursuit of turbocharged splendor, however, please consider the fourth principle of conditioning, *progression*. Dramatic changes via endurance, strength building, and flexibility exercises at desired levels of intensity, frequency, and duration do not occur overnight. Adaptation to muscle-specific overloads takes time. Start at a low level of overload, and gradually increase or progress in exercise intensity and duration. Be sure to build in recovery time. When adaptation occurs in steps, "overload" at the old level is not an overload anymore. This process of increasing levels of overload/adaptation continues as you progress over time to advanced stages of superior fitness approximating your potentials.

You have completed one half the program. You know

more about physical fitness than the next 1,000 or so people you will pass on the streets. Congratulations on your progress. Next week, there will be more on fitness called wellness vital signs, but for now, rest on your laurels.

Check Day Seven. Good work.

Sometimes, efforts to get others to change go awry. Here are two cases of failure from my files:

"I used to chew my nails. I worried that it would ruin my teeth. So, I switched to toothpicks. And got Dutch Elm Disease."

"I read so much about the hazards of smoking that I decided to give up reading."

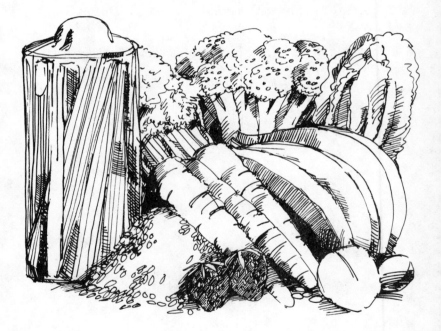

Day Eight

Eat For Performance As Well As Enjoyment

Purpose: In another fifteen minutes (or so), you should have a good appreciation of varied food patterns, basic principles for wellness dining, and a renewed interest in discovering your own approaches to food that help you think and function at your best. You will also be introduced to six ways people eat, only one of which is recommended.

This Day will take more than fifteen minutes to complete. It may take two fifteen-minute sessions. (Let us not be rigid!) It could not be helped. It is not that nutritional awareness is more important than the other four wellness dimensions, nor am I implying that Day Eight is of greater significance than any of the other thirteen Days. There is just a lot of turf to cover when discussing such popular, controversial, and complex matters as food patterns, diets, and all the rest surrounding this subject area.

MOTIVES FOR FOOD CHOICES

There are six kinds of eaters in affluent parts of Western cultures: survivors, vaudevillers, disease avoiders, food faddists, fat fighters, and health enhancers. A word about each is in order.

Survivors eat to stay alive. They would not eat at all if they did not have to. Food is not a high priority with this nothing-for-lunch bunch. These people are simply uninterested in spending time thinking about food or eating. Basically, they eat just about whatever finds its way to their plates, while thinking about something (anything) else. Food bores them; nutrition is of little interest. There are not a lot of survivor eaters.

Vaudevillers are the overwhelming majority of eaters. In this case, food is seen and experienced as entertainment. The emphasis is on how it tastes — period. Nutritional considerations, body-shape implications, the mood of the diner, the source, and the methods of delivery — forget it. All that matters is how it looks, smells, tastes, and feels going down the gullet. Vaudevillers account for the popularity of junk food. For these folks, mealtimes are the high spots of the day. They get up early for breakfast, then start thinking about lunch and supper. The evening meal is the major event of the night, followed in importance only by the midnight snack.

Disease avoiders are the products of health educators, cardiologists, diet authors, and nutritionists. They worry a lot about food. They are obsessed with "scare" research linking one more disease with yet another food they love but henceforth must avoid. They comprise the vast number of persons who try to eat only those foods that have not been identified as possible carcinogens. Thus, their food choices are rather limited. (These folks fret a lot about the health of Canadian rats!) They constantly wonder what kind of edible goody will be their eventual undoing.

Fat fighters are the unhappiest of eaters. They, like the vaudevillers, love to be entertained by food. However, though they may eat more of it, they enjoy it a lot less. Everything they eat turns to hideous adipose (fatty) tissue, or so they believe. Food is associated with guilt, shame, and pounds. Fat fighters spend a lot of money on diet books, spas, doctors and, naturally, restaurants and supermarkets. For them, food is a four-letter word.

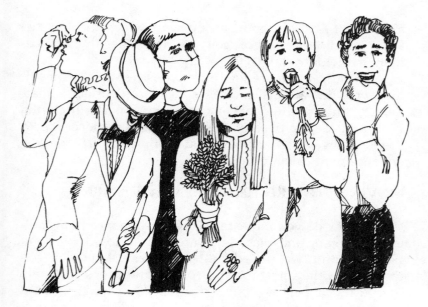

Food faddists are the hardest to take. They want *you* to worry, feel guilty, or get angry about food. If it's not organic, home-grown, or purchased in a "health" food store, it's probably about as good for you as PCB, the food faddists maintain. There are lots of food faddists in California. One friend of mine gets erotic about the subject — he has installed a mirror over his stove (you know, so he can look up at his food and get aroused). A woman friend takes megadoses of Geritol. She mixes the stuff in a blender with wheat germ, Valium, and bone meal. Her blood's so iron-rich she attaches her earrings with magnets.

Health enhancers are the small but growing band of individuals who eat for health, enjoyment, and performance. They are as concerned about, and interested in, the quality and atmosphere (internal and external) of the nutritional experience as the taste. These are the wellness eaters.

This Day is addressed to followers of all six patterns. However, it should help you become a member of the Health Enhancers' Dining Association. (Though non-

existent, it is still a good group with which to identify.)
From a wellness point of view, eating for health enhancement is the only way to fly.

Naturally, there are few pure types; we all at times fit
into survivor, vaudeville, disease-avoider, food-faddist, fat-
fighter, and health-enhancement categories. The trick, the
goal, and the purpose of this Day is to convince you to
spend more of your food-related time in the health-
enhancement category.

MOVING TOWARD HEALTH ENHANCEMENT

So, how do you move to the health-enhancement category? The starting place is awareness of "desirable food
patterns" and "wellness dining principles." After that, you
must begin the quest for your own approaches that help
you be at your best as often as possible. How well off would
you be if you were hailed as North America's greatest
theoretical biochemist, Earth's supreme authority on whole
grains, and the galaxy's foremost expert on food additives,
vitamin supplements, fasting, and colonic irrigation — if
you were not enjoying food and optimal body performance? Not well off. Knowledge without action gets you
close to nowhere at all.

This Day is devoted to a quick summary of nutritional
awareness from the positive side of the dimension. The
ultimate purpose is not to convey nutritional wisdom. I
would like to do a little of that, but the main object is to
motivate you to motivate yourself to pay closer attention to
what there is about food, eating, and the trappings that
adds to, rather than detracts from, health at the pin-
nacle. There is a rich literature on adverse diets and their
valley/pit syndrome of illness consequences. I think you
will be more challenged as well as satisfied to search out
nutritional information focused on the peaks of optimal
functioning. Day Twelve will get you started.

Why So Many Survivors, Vaudevillers, Disease Avoiders, Food Faddists, and Fat Fighters?

The major reasons why so many folks eat poorly and suffer around food are: (1) their parents, mates, and friends eat poorly; (2) the junk food, cattle, and dairy industries are politically powerful, so only the "good news" about their products gets much play; (3) the nutritional experts are, on the whole, conservative "play-it-safe" paralysis-of-analysis types; (4) nutritional information provided in the schools and elsewhere is usually boring, academic, and theoretical, not down-to-earth and practical; (5) the culture does not support wellness food patterns; (6) nutrition seems so incredibly complex; and (7) the positive benefits of nutritional awareness and wellness dining practices have not been studied, described, or widely understood. This last reason for sorry diets is the most important; you can affect this variable more than any of the others.

Just think of the effect that a shift in consciousness from illness avoidance or disease postponement to one of health ennoblement would have on the motivations of fat fighters and disease avoiders. Instead of not eating something (or worrying that something should not be eaten but eating it anyway) because it may cause hoof-and-mouth disease in ten years, people would enjoy food while contemplating the gains it will bring tomorrow! In other words, the motive shifts from not getting something negative in the distant future to anticipating a positive return the next day.

What a superb advantage it is to reach a point where you actually enjoy foods which provide maximum energy, power, balance, recovery, and self-worth. Set this challenge as your goal and you can overcome what your cultures taught you to like that really does not serve your well-being. You do not have to rely on powerful lobbies and special interests, unimaginative nutritionists, the soporific educational system, the negative reinforcements of a nutritionally poisonous culture, or the idea that you need a

Ph.D. in biochemistry or equivalent expertise to be sufficiently informed about the subject of food and sound dietary practices to pursue nutritional wellness.

You need only two fundamental skills to shape your own wellness-oriented nutritional lifestyle: (1) a rudimentary knowledge of nutritional basics — knowing which food types are strengthening and which are debilitating; and (2) an awareness and reorientation of food preference. The information assembled for this Day is designed to help you develop both skills. In addition, you will be greatly advantaged if you cultivate a few attitudes which complement the basic skills. These include a curiosity and interest in pursuing additional knowledge at your own pace, an awareness of how selected foods and eating patterns affect your body, a commitment to conscious and deliberate dining habits, and a confidence in yourself and the way you choose to eat.

The possession of these skills will not mean you know all there is to be discovered about nutrition, that your diet is perfect, that others should eat the way you do, or that you should be teaching the subject. It simply means you are well along your own pathway to a health-enhancing nutritional lifestyle, that you feel good about your food choices, that you are supporting your wellness lifestyle with sound dining, and that you are enjoying truly good food even more than the rank, decaying offal you used to ingest. Ugh!

THE FITNESS CONNECTION

One of the basic notions to understand about nutritional well-being from a health-enhancement perspective is that your level of physical fitness is as important as the kind of food you eat. This is due to the fact that physical activity and fitness levels influence what and how you eat, your digestive process, and the results you get from the food experience. Of course, your position on the nutritional continuum is also greatly affected by your ability to recognize and manage stress, to shape a supportive environment, and to know better than to look only to doctors, drugs or other medical approaches to weight control and good nutrition. For the moment, however, there are good reasons to look closely at the impact of one particular wellness dimension on your nutritional well-being, namely, physical fitness.

To deal with nutrition without considering exercise is like promoting wellness from a physical perspective alone, without recognizing the mental, emotional, spiritual, and societal implications. It would be incomplete, short of its potential. That is why crash diets seldom really work in the short term and never work in the long view. If you diet without exercise, you lose some excess weight *and* lean body or muscle tissue. You do nothing to change basic food and exercise patterns that got you fat in the first place; so your weight goes up and down in roller coaster fashion with one diet after another (termed "the rhythm method of girth control"). Forget the word "diet," which has come to mean a temporary way of eating for weight-control purposes. Concentrate instead on the total connection between fitness and nutrition, and begin to think of ways to develop lifelong food and exercise patterns for optimal well-being. Conditioning and fitness are related more to body-fat/lean-muscle-tissue ratios than to body weight, and it is *exercise* — not food types — that determines whether you develop and maintain a healthy body-fat/lean-muscle ratio (15% fat or less for males, 19% of less for females). The bathroom scale does more harm than good if it gives you a sense that a certain body weight alone is a desirable goal, and leads you to concentrate on calories taken down to the neglect of calories burned up. Fat fighters of the world, unite. Realize that optimal nutrition involves optimal fitness. Separating the two dimensions in Days Seven, Eight, and Twelve is just a necessary device for organizing and presenting a lot of miscellaneous data and viewpoints on each topic. As you read this, recall the distinction between muscle mass and fat, and know that the true challenge is to fashion your physical characteristics (muscle mass, blood chemistry, cell metabolism, etc.) so as to become an efficient "fat converter." Unless you are some kind of a saint, you will not always follow basic wellness food patterns. (I don't, and I am a saint.) Fortunately, if you have superb muscle tone, high metabolism, low body fat, and outstanding cardiovascular endurance and efficiency, chances are that junk-food binges will be less frequent, less desired, and less harmful (if, indeed, there is any adverse effect at all).

So, welcome again to the wonderful world of dining for health enhancement. How you shape your lifestyle in this dimension is affected by, and conditions your role in, the other wellness dimensions.

THE BOTTOM LINE: DINING FOR SUPERHEALTH

The essence of what I believe is foundation knowledge for pursuing a wellness-oriented approach to nutrition can be expressed in one sentence: eat mostly fruits, vegetables (preferably raw and fresh) and whole grains; limit intake of saturated fats and refined sugar, flour, and salt; and avoid foods containing nitrites/nitrates (and other potentially hazardous chemical additives).

For optimal performance, you need an optimal diet. Other things being more or less the same, you do not need salt tablets, vitamin and mineral supplements, added sugar, or temperature extremes. You do need a variety of whole foods or quality calories; a balance between fuel intake (food) and energy burn-up (exercise); favorable daily combinations of water, calories, protein, fats, carbohydrates, minerals, and vitamins; more red blood cells (from increased fitness); extra water (before, during, and after vigorous activity); and fewer inhibiting habits (smoking, alcohol).

Unfortunately, this kind of advice in itself is of limited use to you for a couple reasons: (1) it is based on my experience — reading and listening, and experimenting with agreeable and disagreeable foods — not yours; and (2) it is too packaged and easy — you have to work for and come to value your own "truths" in this regard if a wellness food pattern is going to work for you. A brief discussion of nutrition principles as reference points may help you discover your own unique wellness pathways. Think of these as starting points. The nutrition books listed in the Honor Roll Section are good bets for serious (but not dull) reading on this dimension.

Fruits, Vegetables, and Whole Grains

Complex carbohydrates (e.g., all vegetables and fruits, breads and cereals, dry beans and peas, lentils, nuts and nutlike seeds, peanuts) are the mainstay of a health enhancer's food pattern. You do not have to be a vegetarian to enjoy and flourish on the rich variety of goodies that fall under this broad classification. People who derive all or nearly all of their food energy from such sources (e.g., Seventh Day Adventists) have less body fat, lower levels of blood cholesterol, lower rates of cardiovascular disease, distemper, and so forth. It is generally acknowledged that Americans would be a great deal healthier if they ate more of an assortment of these foods and a lot less of certain others. Doing so involves almost no risks on the down side and exceptional possibilities for improved well-being on the positive side. The issues involved are, however, hotly debated since there are powerful economic and other interests at "steak" (pun intended).

Fruits, vegetables, and whole grains can provide just about everything you need in terms of nutrients, including vitamins, minerals, fiber, protein, fats, and carbohydrates. These foods come in extraordinary varieties, are relatively cheap (in most places), and are delicious — even to the worseness-trained palates deadened by sugars, salts and other aberrations. In short, it is hard to knock fruits, veggies, and whole grains, but it is possible. (After all, what's perfect?) If, for example, you choose to eat *only* fruits, vegetables, and whole grains (no meat, poultry, fish, eggs, or dairy products), you have to know a few rudimentary things about food combinations.

Some dieticians believe that exclusive reliance on fruits, vegetables, and whole grains could lead to protein deficiencies and leave your body short of calcium, folic acid, iron, niacin, ribloflavin, and vitamins B12 and B6. The keys to avoiding such problems are: (1) don't rely exclusively on fruits, vegetables, and whole grains; or (2) if you choose to do so, devote a little extra study to food combining and other considerations discussed in vegetarian-oriented magazines. There are plenty of articles written each month about informed use of cereal products, legumes and flours, and how to obtain 20 essential amino acids from varied protein sources. You can combine foods from plant sources so that the amino-acid deficiencies of one are more than covered by the other. Best sellers have been published in recent years that describe this process in detail (e.g., Frances Moore Lappe's *Diet for a Small Planet*). An example would be to pair, at one meal, cereals and grains (rich in methionine) with legumes, such as peas and beans (rich in lycine), and occasional seeds, nuts and/or food supplements for needed iron, calcium, and B12 (mostly found in meat and dairy products, though soybeans are a nutritious, inexpensive, and complete protein alternative). A two-to-one combination of corn and beans gives you protein superior to meat at about 10 percent the cost. In short, it is easy to understand why a wellness-oriented diner would want to emphasize fruits, vegetables (organic), and whole grains as the mainstay of a sound diet.

As with anything else, organic fruits and vegetables free of chemical residues are best, but it can be an expense and a hassle to pursue this hard-to-prove characteristic. If you have the energy and opportunity to join a food cooperative, to buy direct from aware and conscientious farmers, to pay the more expensive natural-food-store prices, or to grow your own, then, by all means, go for it. If not, do not worry about it. Worrying will get you nowhere worth going.

By the way, you do not have to take bran to school with you every day to be thought of as a regular person. These same complex carbohydrates in vegetables are also high in fiber or roughage which you need for healthful bowel movements. Fiber is the indigestible portion of such veggies and fruits as carrots, celery, and apples. In the large bowel, fiber absorbs water and makes stools larger, softer, and heavier, thereby speeding the passage of wastes through the digestive tract. Thus, you not only avoid grim problems as you grow older (e.g., hemorrhoids, diverticulitis, and so on), but, more important, you get to enjoy the experience of full and invigorating excretory functions several times a day. Functions which must be performed should be enjoyed.

Do the vegetables and fruits look fresh? You do not have to be the green grocer or head of the produce section in a supermarket to know quality when you see it. While U.S. Department of Agriculture studies* show that, under reasonable conditions of distribution and marketing, loss of vitamin C rarely exceeds 10 percent. The picture looks quite different for fruits and vegetables without a thick skin. Leafy vegetables, for example, deteriorate in quality and appearance rather quickly. If the lettuce does not look too spiffy, it probably is not much of a nutrient bargain either. In addition, since most of these foods have already been out of the ground or off the trees for a week or more in the journey to the store and then to you, it's better to enjoy them immediately and shop more often than to keep fruits and veggies around for a week or more. As for obtaining the ultimate in nutrient content, try to experience a tomato right off the vine or an apple from a tree. In taste and food value,

---

*John Korchta and Bernard Feinberg, "Effect of Harvesting and Handling on Nutrient Composition of Fruits and Vegetables," (U.S. Department of Agriculture: Washington, D.C., 1979).

there is no comparison with the store-bought variety. So, let your eyeball be your guide.

The "whole-grain" issue is one with which you should be familiar. There are good reasons, from the food processors' perspective, for dissecting the grains (shelf life, profits) — but few good reasons for you to buy the stuff. When the fibrous outer layer of the wheat (or bran) and the vitamin-rich inner kernel (or germ) are removed, and when the remainder is bleached, milled, and sifted, there is not much left. Gone are most of the roughage, B vitamins, vitamin E, and the essential trace minerals — zinc, magnesium, chromium, and manganese. True, the process of enrichment returns a few of the nutrients, but the result is a poorer quality flour than if the wheat had been left whole in the first place. It is like being mugged of your bike but given bus fare home. Here is a chart that makes the point.

COMPARISON OF SEVEN BASIC
NUTRIENTS IN WHEAT FLOUR (PER POUND)*

	Unenriched	Enriched	Whole Wheat
Protein (gms)	47.6	47.6	60.3
Fat (mgs)	4.5	4.5	9.1
Calcium (mgs)	73	73	186
Iron (mgs)	3.6	13.0-16.5	15.0
Thiamine (mgs)	.28	2.9	2.49
Riboflavin (mgs)	.21	1.8	.54
Niacin (mgs)	4.1	24.0	19.7

It is worth the extra effort to buy whole-wheat bread, millet, nonsugary granola made with whole grains, brown rice, bulgur wheat, buckwheat, barley, corn, legumes, oats, and other foods with natural roughage. You do not have to

---

*Source: Nutritive Value of American Foods, (U.S. Department of Agriculture, Handbook No. 456: Washington, D.C., November, 1975).

be hung up on disease avoidance to appreciate the value and advantages of dietary fiber for digestive regularity. Ever try meditating, dancing, jogging, or making love while constipated? Very uncomfortable and distracting.

Of course, anything can be overdone. I know a doctor in Miami who told me about a patient who called her early one morning to demand that she prescribe something for his regularity: "Doctor, I have a terrible problem. I eat lots of whole grains and I have a bowel movement every morning at 6:00 A.M.!" The physician said, "I can't be sympathetic. Why do you bother me with such a so-called problem. You should be happy — half my patients would like to be in your situation. Keep eating whole grains, by all means. By the way, why *do* you consider this a problem?" The patient responded, "Because I don't get up until 7:00."

Controlled Intake of Saturated Fats — The Meat Issue

Putting aside the moral, ethical (i.e., world hunger and the fact that 21 pounds of plant protein are invested for every pound of edible meat protein we get back from the animal), and economic (i.e., meat is very expensive to buy) reasons for eating little or no animal protein, there is another good reason to eschew (rather than to chew) most or all meat products: they are loaded with saturated fat. Saturated fat, the kind that is hard at room temperature, has been implicated as a villain in just about every degenerative disease named in modern times — all of which not only wipe you out before your time, but also slow you down during your stay on Earth. Therefore, the real hazard in consuming excess saturated fat is not related to longevity; the true concern is with quality and physical excellence. Remember, the nasty disease manifestations are only end-states of conditions that build up over long periods of time. The true impact of high-fat diets is measured in the extent to which such illness-producing elements slow you down, rob you of power and vitality, and limit the realization of your potentials.

To eat, or not to eat, meat products — that is the question. Some meats are relatively lean (e.g., turkey, chicken, veal), but nearly all "red" meats such as beef, pork, lamb, etc., are very high in saturated fat. What to do? Well, there are, to be sure, good reasons for consuming meat: it is the third best protein source (after eggs and milk); it is rich in certain B vitamins; it tastes great (if, like most of us, you have developed a taste for fat); it is fashionable and/or convenient to do so in most cultures; and cutting and chewing on it may, suggests Jean Mayer, president of Tufts University and a well-known nutritionist, help you feel macho. (Mayer suggests that desk-bound males get reassurance regarding their masculinity by eating red meat and that it is "the motorcycle of the middle-aged.") Unfortunately, the extremely high saturated fat content in meat (a "choice grade of cooked and trimmed sirloin steak is still 50 percent fat) creates serious problems for the steak-and-potatoes-for-lunch bunch. According to a Senate Committee report, the average American obtains 42 percent of his/her calories from fat sources — which nearly everyone agrees is conducive to obesity in particular and premature worseness in general. But the high fat content of meat is just part of the problem with eating meat regularly. American meat contains high levels of antibiotics, hormones, and pesticide residues. If this were not a health-enhancement book, I would describe the situation with one drug called diethylstilbestrol (DES), a synthetic chemical used to fatten cattle. But who needs scare tactics — the main problem with meat eating is that it is not associated with optimal states of health. In fact, the Institute of Health Research in San Francisco, an organization that has been conducting longitudinal studies of blood composition in different population groups for years, claims that the healthiest blood chemistries in their research findings belong to vegetarian runners, followed by sedentary vegetarians, followed by meat-eating runners. No need to do anything drastic in the near term, however. Just pay attention to how your body feels after ingesting red meats, if you choose to do so, and read up on the issues at your leisure. For purposes of limiting saturated fat intake alone, it makes sense to know the issues and make your own informed decisions.

It is not sufficient to simply reduce the amount of saturated fat in your diet. One must also pay attention to the quality of the vegetable fat (which is mostly unsaturated) that one consumes. All margarines, Crisco, and most oils on your grocer's shelves are hydrogenated. This process changes the chemical structure of the oil to something which the body is not used to. The effects of this change have only recently been studied, and the preliminary results indicate that the changes are not good for the body. As an alternative, consider using cold-pressed, unrefined vegetable polyunsaturated form (except palm and coconut oils, which are mostly saturated). They are processed with a minimum of heat, without chemical solvents, and without mineral-removing filtering.

Since the concern of this Day is optimal performance, a few words are in order about the connections between high-fat diets and the body's ability to utilize oxygen — the basis of high performance in any physical activity.

A number of scientists have speculated on the effects of byproducts of metabolism known as free radicals. These are often very small, broken-off bits of oxygen molecules that do not fire properly, which damages vital cell membranes. Any excess of free radicals in and around cells may be responsible for both disease and premature aging (or poor functioning).

Refined Sugar

You do not need a wellness book to learn that refined sugar is far and away the most abused drug in America (125 lbs. per person annually), and many believe, the deadliest.

Chances are excellent that you know this. I will not dwell on all the ghastly conditions that result from thinking that a six-course gourmet treat consists of five Hostess Twinkies and a Coke, or six supergoops dipped in chocolate fudge.

You can get away with sugar loading for a long time — if you chose your parents wisely, and you have a super pancreas and all kinds of other physiological advantages going for you. If your motivation was only to avoid worseness conditions, it would be hard to resist eating globs of sugar like everyone else. After all, the stuff does taste great; it's addictive; it's available everywhere; and it seems to give an immediate and pleasurable energy lift. Fortunately, you would not be reading a wellness book if your motivation was to avoid or prevent disease, so you probably are interested in the effects of sugar on optimal functioning. In this respect, refined sugar is a disaster. Briefly, it is high in calories but devoid of nutrients. In fact, not only is it without vitamins and minerals but worse, it robs the body of other nutrients (B vitamins) in order to metabolize the stuff. Refined sugar (or honey, molasses, brown, raw, or turbanado sugar) is rapidly absorbed into the bloodstream; the pancreas has to produce an insulin shot to lower blood-sugar levels. Large quantities of the stuff taken day after day upset the delicate balance of glucose (blood sugar) and insulin. The temporary high quickly becomes a longer lasting low. How can you pursue your best potentials for well-being when you are disoriented, dizzy, or worse? A low blood-sugar condition is called "hypoglycemia," the symptoms of which are bizarre behavior, indecision, impotence, depression, and other characteristics of low-level worseness. If two teaspoonful of sugar circulating in the blood are normal, and 20 teaspoonful are the current average levels,* then it is no wonder that so many zanies are out and about.

Sugar-laden products come in many forms, not all of

*"Low Blood Sugar Can Get You Fired," *Executive Fitness Newsletter* (March 10, 1979), p. 2.

which are obvious. For example, snacks such as crackers and breakfast foods, salad dressing, ketchup, and most other processed foods have immoderate amounts of refined sugar thrown in for "taste" purposes. Here is a sampling of foods with the percent of sugar listed to give you the idea:

PERCENTAGE OF SUGAR IN COMMON FOODS

Sugar of all varieties including corn syrup, honey, sucrose, and sugars in fruit and vegetables.

Wish Bone Italian Dressing	7.3%
Coca-Cola	8.9%
Skippy Peanut Butter	9.2%
Ritz Crackers	11.8%
Wyler's beef flavor bouillon cubes	14.8%
Cool Whip	21.0%
Sealtest Chocolate Ice Cream	21.4%
Hamburger Helper	23.0%
Quaker 100% Natural Cereal	23.9%
Heinz Tomato Ketchup	28.9%
Wish Bone Russian Dressing	30.2%
Shake'n Bake Barbecue Style	50.9%
Hershey's Milk Chocolate Candy Bar	51.4%
Coffee-mate Non-Dairy Creamer	65.4%
Jell-o (cherry flavor)	82.6%

From *Consumer Reports,* March 1978.

So how do you kick the habit, or at least keep it from hindering your pursuit of higher possibilities? No easy answers, as usual. Awareness helps; vigilance seems essential. Even small changes constitute progress.

Salt and Other Marginal Products

The average American gets about 12 grams of salt daily; most research suggests we can do nicely with less than three grams per day. Excessive salt intake creates circulatory-system problems, and salt abuses are linked with high blood pressure, heart disease, kidney failure, and so on. As with sugar, cultural norms set us up to add salt to foods in order to "zing" bored taste buds. It is worth the effort to de-program a salt habit. Try a few alternatives. I managed, over time, to eliminate salt by experimenting with alternatives like miso, soy sauce, natural salad dressings, lemon juice, sea veggies (e.g., kelp powder), and countless varieties of herbs. Now I have to work on discovering the hidden salts added *for* me by the manufacturers. This is the *real* challenge. Take a look at the sodium content per serving of a few popular foods.

SODIUM IN COMMON FOODS

Food	Amount	Sodium in Milligrams*
McDonald's Big Mac	1	1510
Soy sauce (about 20% salt)	1 tablespoon	1320
Chef Boy-ar-dee Beefaroni	7.5 ounces	1186
Swanson's Fried Chicken Dinner	1 dinner	1152
Campbell's Beans and Franks	8 ounces	958
Campbell's tomato soup	10 ounces	950
McDonald's Egg McMuffin	1	914
Herb-Ox Instant Broth	1 packet	818
Corned Beef, cooked	3 ounces	800
Oscar Mayer Bologna	3 slices	672
Ham, cooked	3 ounces	636
Creamed Cottage Cheese	1 cup	580
Green Olives	5 small (½ ounce)	345
Celeste Frozen Pizza	2 ounces	328
Wishbone Italian Dressing	1 tablespoon	315
Oscar Mayer Bacon	3 slices	302
Ritz Crackers	9	288
Kellogg's Cornflakes	1 ounce	260
Hostess Twinkies	1	240
Kraft Process American Cheese	1 ounce	238

*Sodium values for brand-name products were determined by Consumers Union (*Consumers Reports,* March 1979) and Center for Science in the Public Interest (*Nutrition Action,* March 1978). The other values are from Agriculture Handbook No. 456, *Nutritive Value of American Foods in Common Units.*

Pillsbury Sugar Cookies	3	210
Potato Chips	14 chips	191
Kraft Cheddar Cheese	1 ounce	190
Popcorn, salted	1 cup	175
Catsup	1 tablespoon	155
Mayonnaise	1 tablespoon	130
Peanut Butter	1 tablespoon	97
Mustard, prepared	1 teaspoon	65
Salted Peanuts	1 tablespoon	38

Coffee. An average size cup contains 100 mg. of caffeine — a stimulant not designed to help you maintain your equilibrium and relaxed balance. Since 250 mg. will raise your adrenalin and blood-pressure levels temporarily, then drop you like a rock, it is not an optimal product for wellness purposes. If you like the taste, try herbal teas or a coffee substitute made of all natural ingredients, such as malted barley, chicory, and rye (e.g., cafix, Postum). I have been working on this for six years, and I am down to a cup a day. Unfortunately, I still really like the stuff. I rationalize that one cup will not hurt or hinder me. I realize it is a weak justification. I'll keep trying.

Ice cream. Delicious stuff, but unfortunately, it has become a landfill for all kinds of non-nutritive chemicals, including colorings, stabilizers, flavorings, emulsifiers, preservatives, additives, and last and least (in quality, not quantity), refined sugar. Maybe you can find a distributor of a somewhat unchemicalized, moderately sweetened ice cream, or perhaps you will experiment with making your own. Where I live, there are several "natural" ice cream manufacturers, but the cost is greater and the taste is different from what my own children expect. (They do not worry about the cost when Dad treats, but they are not used to the "icy" quality and do not like it as well. In addition, the natural store does not have chocolate "jimmies" in which to dip the ice cream — or sugar cones!) As with everything else, changes in old taste habits are gradual, at best. The partial challenge is to find a natural ice cream that tastes better than the artificial brand X glop, and which is widely available at comparable prices. The whole challenge is to decide you don't like the stuff anymore.

Soft Drinks. The scourge of the earth. Most have about nine teaspoons of sugar per 12-ounce serving, and enough chemicals to build a Frankenstein. Leave it for the monster — or your hair will fall out and your eyes will cross. Unfortunately, a lot of people are not leaving it for the monster. Sodas have surpassed coffee as America's most popular drink. In 1979, they accounted for a third of the U.S. beverage dollar; the average person drank 410 12-ounce soft drinks last year. (Source: Nutrition Action, August, 1981, p. 8.)

Given all the evidence and the weight of opinion concerning the illness-causing properties of soft drinks, ice cream, coffee, salt, refined sugar, red meat, and devitalized grains, it is easy to see why so many belong to the disease-avoider society of worried eaters. It is a relief to have a health-enhancement alternative just to get your mind off all these food hazards.

Eggs. The controversy about eggs centers on their high cholesterol content, which for some (mostly older, sedentary) people is a problem. However, recent studies show little or no effect on the serum-cholesterol levels of active people — such as yourself — who pursue wellness lifestyles. So, unless you suspect a problem or know of one from blood tests, worry not. Eggs are an easy-to-assimilate, high-quality, complete protein source. I would say "eat and be merry," save for another problem: the residues in eggs from the chemicals fed to hens. I do not know if you have ever seen a chicken factory, but it ain't pretty. The little creatures (called "beasties" by the late Dr. Halbert L. Dunn) never touch the ground, see the light of day, or get any exercise. I do not know how chickens feel about this, but I suspect that this unnatural situation has an effect on the quality of the poultry and eggs that end up on our plates. Take your chances or look into it, and consider buying eggs from reputable natural food stores or rural stores supplied by farmers where the "beasties" have a better life and thus are likely to be better for you.

Milk and Milk Products. It is not true that everybody needs milk, as the dairy industry would have you believe. Lots of bodies, my own included, do well on milk (skim only); many enjoy it, but about 15 percent of white and 20 percent of all black people tested in a John Hopkins University study proved unable to digest milk lactose. Milk is a good source of vitamin A, phosphorus, riboflavin, B12, folacin, calcium, magnesium, and protein, but that is of little consequence if you do not have lactose, the digestive enzyme for breaking down milk sugar or lactose.

Whole milk is a questionable item even if you have, as most Americans do, the ability to digest milk properly. A cup of whole milk contains 10 grams of fat. It is unlikely that any of us needs four glasses of milk daily, as the milk industry has suggested. The link between milk consumption and calcium sufficiency is probably another milk-industry hype. Some recent studies have shown no relationship between calcium intake and bone thickness. Furthermore, calcium is widely available in other sources which are more digestible, such as whole-grain cereals, broccoli, chard, greens, and artichokes. Consider switching to skim milk (only half the calorie content of whole milk and none of the fat) and other dairy products such as low-fat cottage cheese, kefir, buttermilk, low-fat cheeses, and powdered milk. All of these have fewer calories and little or no saturated fat.

Alcohol. Alcohol is a drug. It depresses the central nervous system. Even small quantities adversely affect the finer movements of physical coordination. Your decision regarding when to use it, if at all, should be influenced as much by your interest in and commitment to physical excellence as by the momentary pressures and opportunities.

Smoking. Perverse as it is to list this foul and utterly pornographic habit with nutritional considerations, I mention it at this point because: (1) it is an oral gratification; (2) it is frequently practiced at mealtimes; (3) it is a marginal product; and (4) it interferes with the body's use of certain nutrients and limits oxygen consumption and utilization. No point in listing all the diseases with which the smoker plays Russian roulette, the added sick days, lowered life expectancy, bad breath, and all the other negatives associated with having a weed containing 4,000 compounds sticking in your face. There is one basis for not smoking and avoiding those who do that alone should be sufficient for anyone pursuing a wellness lifestyle — smoking inhibits upward direction and continued progress toward your own best potentials for well-being. Just thinking about this excrescence makes me cough.

Additives. You have surely heard enough about all the varied forms of leprosy, cancer, hangnails, and other unpleasant illnesses associated with the 2,700 or so additives in our food for purposes of preservation and to affect taste, texture, and appearance. Considering that another 10,000 substances unintentionally taint our foods, including residues of pesticides and herbicides and leaching from packaged materials, it is clear that we are getting more than we bargain for in supermarkets. The list includes, but is not limited to, leavening agents (e.g., baking powder) to get a rise out of baked goods, glazing agents to make surfaces shiny, anti-foaming agents in order that containers can be filled, foaming agents for bubbles, emulsifiers for light texture and mixing, firming agents for added body during canning, thickeners to prevent ice-crystal formation in frozen goods, and artificial coloring agents for sense appeal. No point in worrying about all this, but it would not hurt to make some effort to try to buy less processed foods, grow a little of your own, know your sources and read labels. (If you cannot pronounce an ingredient, it is probably not good for you. Not very scientific, but probably basically true!) MSG (monosodium glutamate), for example, is a hazard found in Chinese restaurants. Derived from wheat or corn gluten or sugar beet byproducts, it is considered a "flavor enhancer." More often, it gives people an allergic headache, nausea, or general feeling of disequilibrium. I always ask that it be left out when I visit Chinese restaurants. You cannot avoid some additives some of the time if you live in or near the big cities (or small towns either), but you can minimize the "chemical feast" characteristics of the modern food supply by being conscious of the most flagrant abuses by the processors. If you avoid processed meats and junk food, read labels, and enjoy complex carbohydrates (no easy task at first), you will be well on your way to controlling the additive problem.

Nitrates and Nitrites and Other Additives

Sodium nitrite and nitrate, which the pork and other meat industries have legally added to their products (in amounts of up to 200 and 300 parts per million, respectively) for decades, may not cause or contribute to cancer or otherwise disturb our delicate biological systems. The debate, while heated, is made complex by conflicting research results and the varied interpretations of the studies. But one thing is certain: nobody has ever made a good case that nitrites and nitrates do anything *positive* for you. Why turn your body into a little laboratory for the pork and related industries? Just thinking about what these people do to hot dogs, bologna, and other meat byproducts gives me a mild attack of botulism.

OTHER CONSIDERATIONS

As you become more involved in and satisfied with conscious food choices that complement your evolving wellness lifestyle, you will hear a lot about three issues dear to the heart of every food faddist: supplements, fasting, and diets. A comment or two on each seems in order, though I encourage you to read or at least skim one or two of the hundreds of books readily available on each of the subjects.

Supplements. Whether or not to pop vitamin/mineral tablets on a regular basis is, like everything else, something you have to decide. This debate has not been settled in my time, and probably will not be in yours, either. Which vitamins and minerals to take, how often, in what dosage, for what purposes, in synthetic or "natural" forms, and so on — the range of issues is extensive. Fortunately or not, there is no shortage of experts ready and willing to give you detailed answers on what you should do regarding all of these issues, and more. You can choose your expert (or food guru) or consider varied points of view — and then shape your own.

There are two reasons for taking supplements: to avoid deficiency diseases and to enable optimal functioning. The different goals are of profound consequence: for example, the amount of vitamin C required by one person to prevent scurvy and the amount needed by another for optimal cellular functioning is quite different. Only a few supplement advocates emphasize the latter — the system is focused on the former (a close parallel to the way it is with the so-called "health system," which in fact ignores health in favor of disease/illness treatment and symptom alleviation). Regarding deficiency avoidance, there is evidence that some people (certain pregnant or menstruating women) have insufficient iron intake, and preschoolers and many others do not always obtain even the marginal RDA (recommended daily allowance) levels established by the federal government. This, of course, is no surprise when consideration is given to the effects of high-calorie, low-nutrient junk foods which are the staples of large numbers of Americans of all ages.

Another problem, from the deficiency perspective, is that many foods are grown in mineral-poor soils and polluted air, and plants are often picked short of maturity, damaged in transit to the marketplace, and cooked to excess — all of which drain nutrients. In addition, our needs vary — some have inherited weaknesses, others strengths; some thrive on stress, others suffer; and some are better at eliminating cellular wastes than others. In short, we vary — as do our minimum requirements. Personally, I believe it is not difficult to obtain all the vitamins and minerals you need from the foods you eat, most of the time. Even a wellness diner, however, experiences situations when supplements may be a reasonably good bet — for example, extra vitamin C when under high stress, or possibly when feeling the effects of a cold, or when travel or other conditions have adversely affected your normal food pattern. Even in such cases, the supplement(s) will not be a sure thing, but is not likely to do any harm if megadoses are avoided. I occasionally take a gram of vitamin C and/or a multivitamin/mineral supplement, but for the most part rely on good food selection as the best source of needed nutrients. Not a lot is known about taking supplements for optimal functioning, as opposed to avoiding deficiencies. If it could be proven that bone meal would help me run the marathon in less than two hours and 35 minutes, or become a sexual acrobat at age 100, I would be first in line for a large supply. Given how things are, I'll continue to place reliance on good food for the nutrients I need. Whatever you do, try to stay open to (and reasonably critical in assessing) new information.

If you are going to take supplements, take them with meals for better nutrient assimilation and utilization. Never let food supplements become a substitute for varied and balanced foods, and check if the supplement you do use is worth the effort (and cost). Some are not well balanced, in that they contain large amounts of cheapo vitamins (e.g., pyridoxine). Dr. Roger Williams, the head of the Clayton Foundation Biochemical Institute, has suggested minimum vitamin- and mineral-content standards for multipurpose supplements.

You might want to check the label on your own brand to see how it stands up to this criterion of adequacy.

VITAMINS		MINERALS	
Vitamin A	10,000 units	Calcium	300.0 mg.
Vitamin D	500 units	Phosphate	250.0 units
Ascorbic Acid (Vit. C)	100 mg.	Magnesium	100.0 mg.
Thiamine (Vit. B₁)	2 mg.	Cobalt	0.1 mg.
Riboflavin (Vit. B₂)	2 mg.	Copper	1.0 mg.
Pyridoxine (Vit. B₆)	3 mg.	Iodine	0.1 mg.
Niacinamide	20 mg.	Iron	10.0 mg.
Pantothenate	20 mg.	Manganese	1.0 mg.
Vitamin B₁₂	5 mg.	Molybdenum	0.2 mg.
Tocopherols (Vit. E)	5 mg.	Zinc	5.0 mg.
Inositol	100 mg.		
Choline	100 mg.		

Source: Dr. Roger Williams

Finally, resist the temptation to treat an illness or disease with high doses of vitamin/mineral supplements, without discussing your ideas (or the research promises you read about) with a number of nutritionally-informed physicians. Suppose you read that sexual research with rats at the Mayo Clinic seems to indicate that high intake of vitamin E improves both the potency and lusts of the test subjects. What do you make of that? Simple. If you're a rat, vitamin E might help you out.

Fasting. There are intriguing as well as outrageous claims made for and against fasting. The proponents are the health food and holistic health set; the detractors are led by M.D.s and nutritionists. The first group describes fasting in euphoric terms and believes the practice results in crashing insights, wondrous and multiple orgasms, and communications with the gods (not to dwell upon the alleged benefits of clean bowels — enemas are very popular among the fasting advocates); the second group describes fasting as a dangerous gimmick, and claims that weight losses are almost always short-lived. So, what is the real truth? It might be useful to sketch in brief what happens during a period of extended non-eating. Basically, if the body has fewer calories than it needs, it will burn stored fat (another way to state the process is that the body eats itself during a fast). Instead of converting the carbohydrate glucose and other fuel, the body burns liver glucoses and muscle proteins. This process causes large salt and water losses and leads to the breakdown of fat compounds in the liver (called ketones), which go into the bloodstream and are oxidized by enzymes in the brain. The oxidation of ketones, occurring about one week into a fast, becomes the body's main energy source. As you can sense from this sketchy summary of what's happening during a fast, there are protein losses, which means that muscle and other tissues are at risk if the body is not supplemented with some kind of glucose, minerals, and amino acid sources. Another problem is a build-up of uric acid, which can crystallize as kidney or bladder stones if insufficient water or other liquid is not taken daily (two quarts). All of which is mentioned not to discourage fasting — it might be good for you — but to emphasize that the body is a wondrous and complex organism designed to work well. Is it really necessary to screw around with a good thing and risk voiding nature's warranty? Perhaps, in certain circumstances for special purposes and under qualified supervision, it may be helpful to try an extended (more than one day) fast. As always, you have to decide. If the benefits of fasting were 10 percent of what advocates claim — (weight loss, energy abundance, disease prevention and cures, spiritual enlightenment, reverse or slowing of the aging process, reduced sleep requirements, elimination of alcoholism, smoking, and other antisocial behaviors, universal harmony between men and women, and so on) — it ought to be required by law! But these and other claims have not been documented by impartial observers, and thus some reserve may be well advised. If abused, an extended and uninformed fast could literally be your "ultimate" or "last chance" diet! One thing seems certain: a fast is no substitute for an awareness of nutritional principles combined with regular aerobic exercise, controlled and managed stress levels, satisfaction with life purposes, and an appreciation for personal accountability for what goes well or poorly. Weight problems, as with stress, sedentary habits, and other problems, are not amenable to magic bullets or quick cures. Too many people use a fast as if it were a Valium tablet to a happy and meaningful existence, and it becomes just another substitute for undermining lifestyle reform.

Personally, I think there is much to be said for occasional one-day fasts. I periodically abstain from food for a day, not for weight-loss purposes but to demonstrate to myself a certain control over the lure of food. A day without food is a liberating experience — I enjoy the realization that I can suppress food desires for a day. I also like the extra time available when free from planning, obtaining, preparing, eating, and cleaning up after meals.

Diets. Quick weight-loss plans sell more books than sex, and almost always do a lot less good and provide fewer satisfactions for everyone involved. No matter what you like to eat, there is probably a physician or other nutrition "expert" who has written a best seller to the effect that you can eat more of it, or that you can lose weight effortlessly and eat to your heart's content if you buy his program. Well, that is a little exaggerated, but not greatly. Millions of Americans truly are practicing rhythm methods of girth control, losing (and regaining) hundreds and sometimes thousands of pounds in their lifetimes while failing to maintain an optimum weight for living a full and satisfying existence. There are diets for brown rice, grapefruit, caviar (tough if you are on a budget), red meat, anything with fiber, sardines, eggs, milk, and so on. There are high fat/low fat, high carbohydrate/low carbohydrate, and high protein/

low protein diets, and one best-selling M.D.'s ploy that lets "you eat as much as you want, as often as you want." So, who is putting on whom? What is a good diet from a wellness perspective? I suspect you know the answer to this one — that there is no such thing as a good diet, if diet is construed in the popular sense of the word as a temporary food pattern for weight loss (or gain) purposes. As noted above, the best way to control weight is to develop an appreciation for the positive gains of a wellness lifestyle. It is far better to find satisfaction in shaping permanent approaches based on your own nutritional values, preferences and needs, balanced with an awareness of wellness fundamentals in the other dimensions. Diets alone do more harm than good, and rarely work in the long term.

There is more to food than what you eat: before concluding this chapter, it makes sense to give some attention to the how and why of the nutritional experience.

AWARENESS AND REORIENTATION OF FOOD PREFERENCES

Wouldn't it be fine if you only liked those foods that complemented a wellness lifestyle? And, wouldn't it be great to dislike foods loaded with fat, sugar, and all kinds of additives. It would be, and it can be that way, with a little practice and attention to a few techniques for awareness and redirection. The first step is to notice your mood.

I always pass out fresh carrot slices at wellness seminars. I ask people to experience the carrot slice but not to bite into it. I encourage the audience to use their imaginations in becoming fully aware of their response to and enjoyment of the carrot. Short of eating it, I ask them to observe and appreciate the carrot with all their senses. They are encouraged to note the color, texture, and aroma of the carrot slice, to reflect on the carrot growth cycle, and the effects of soils, air, and sun on its quality and availability. They are encouraged to lick the carrot, to rub it against their lips, in short, to "get it on" with the carrot (without actually biting or chewing). While this is taking place, I'm running off data concerning the vitamin and mineral composition of carrots, their high-fiber content, low-calorie characteristic ("Only 20 calories versus 80 in an apple — switch to a carrot a day to keep the doctor away and you will save five pounds in a year"), leading carrot-growing states, multiple uses (e.g., color in salads and moisture to baked goods), and even carrot jokes ("Too many carrots will cause insomnia — your night vision will be so acute you will see through your eyelids, thus having to watch shadows on the bedroom ceiling. Or look at yourself in the mirrors.").

The point of this three- or four-minute carrot game is to enable participants to reflect on the extent to which they can relate to food without immediately consuming it. Large numbers of people use food as entertainment to an excessive degree, and find it maddening to refrain from eating the carrot before the end of the game. Eventually they get to bite the carrot — but to delay chewing for a few moments; then to chew without swallowing; and finally to swallow — being aware of sensations at each stage of the process. Seminar participants are given guidelines by which they can assess the extent to which they may be unconsciously using food for substitute gratification, and ways to interpret their feelings during the carrot game. The Zen or "inner game" of eating a carrot is, of course, just a fun way to get across the idea that how you eat is as important as what you eat. Emotional feelings affect the extent to which you can obtain all the nutrients available in given foods during the digestive process, and these reactions in turn have an influence on the kinds of foods you select and where you shop.

Make an effort to become more aware of how you respond to food, your moods at mealtimes, your motives for eating at a particular moment, why you choose certain foods, and whether you can slow down and be reflective during meal hours. Preface meals with a brief quiet period

— a moment to reflect, whether through prayer, meditation, holding hands or other communion ritual with others, or whatever. Be relaxed when you eat, take time to observe and appreciate the food, and to truly taste each morsel as it is chewed and swallowed. When you eat rapidly, the stomach does not have enough time to sense the presence of food and to signal the "appestat" in the brain that hunger needs have been attended — so you end up overeating. Another tip — if you chew your food thoroughly the starch begins to digest in the mouth, which facilitates digestion in the stomach. Also notice if you are a "polyphasic diner," that is, engaged in other activities while eating — watching TV, reading, shaving, talking, or otherwise allowing your awareness to wander from the food before you.

You can make a conscious choice to like or dislike any given food. You have already made unconscious selections; the challenge now is to relearn preferences to complement your nutritional patterns with other aspects of your wellness lifestyle. There is nothing "biological" about your current likes and dislikes — you did not inherit a taste for sugar slurpies and Ding-Dongs. Nothing physiological will get in the way if you decide you want to flip out over raw veggies and fruit juices, for example. If you allow yourself to think that you cannot change, that expectation will make it so; believe that you will enjoy making gradual changes in your preferences and your realizations will follow accordingly. Anticipate the satisfactions to be had in new flavors and sensations; create images in your mind of the growing powers and energies these foods provide; and celebrate the acquisition of new enjoyments and the diminution of old needs (for empty junk and imitation foods that you do not even like anymore).

Keep a one-week log or inventory of food intake and attitudes. Make sure it is a typical week (not one when you will visit Grandmother Walden, the health food nut who runs a berry farm), and do not make any effort to change your usual habits. Record everything, making separate columns for the place, time of day, food items, quantity, mood before and after dining, eating pace, whether there was a quiet time just before the food was taken, and any observations you want to add. To give you an idea of what your log might look like, here is a record of what my own food

A SAMPLE FOOD LOG

July 18, 1981

Place	Time of day	Food	Quantity
home	8:10 am	granola	a large bowl
		orange juice	8 oz.
home	9:30 am	herbal tea	8 oz.
home	11:30 am	grapefruit	1
home	12:30 pm	apple	1
		salad—lots of veggies added	1 bowl
		apple pie	large slice
home	3:15 pm	cafix (coffee substitute)	8 oz.
		apple	1
		yogurt (plain)	8 oz.
home	4:55 pm	apple juice	8 oz.
restaurant	7:15 pm	mineral water	8 oz.
		salad & soup	
		seafood omelette	lrg. dish
home	10:15 pm	apple juice	10 oz.

pattern was on the day I wrote this section of the chapter. (It is definitely not intended as a model of how you should eat; I realize that my food pattern is not and never will be perfect. I'm satisfied with how things are at this time, though I'm open to growth as my preferences change.)

Mood	Pace	Quiet time	Observations
high energy	deliberate	yes	very hungry—just completed 10 mile run
quiet	slow	no	—
reflective	fast	no	absorbed in work
excited	fast	yes	feeling excited
distracted	slow	yes	concentration of feeling lazy
—	fast	no	—
talkative & exuberant	slow/fast alternately	yes	have to work at slowing down food ingestion
calm	slow	yes	very tired

The purpose of the log is to give you a better sense of your food patterns. At some later point, you might want to share it with a wellness-oriented nutritionist for a nutrient analysis. This should include recommendations on percent of calories (versus actual) from protein, fat, and carbohydrates; identification of problem areas; and specific suggestions on meal preparation, recipes, and similar helpful hints. If you think you may want to use your log for this purpose, list the ingredients of all the foods you consume. For example, under apple pie I would have noted that it contained apples, unsweetened fruit-juice concentrate, starch, salt, flavoring, whole-wheat flour, soybean oil, and water. However, the principal reason for the log is not preparation for a professional analysis, but for raising your sensitivity to your own established food patterns. It is common for people to be highly surprised at the results of a week's log. The insights gained from this process can be invaluable in terms of raised awareness and eventual reorientation of food preferences. The log is also a curious and entertaining bit of memorabilia to look back on. You may find yourself thinking, a year or so from now, "Did I really eat that? It is amazing that I'm still alive!"

Develop a generalized one-month food plan. What might you want to do differently in the next few weeks? What modest changes do you think are realistic, if indeed any are necessary, given your current food patterns? Look over your one-week log another time, and add a new page to the back of the log. On this page, sketch, in general terms, new directions that you will explore in the coming months. For example, you might enter phrases similar to the following:

- I'll think of five ways to reduce my intake of refined sugar (e.g., cut down on soda, ice cream, and candies).
- I'll stop eating hot dogs at the ball park — and will instead bring sandwiches from the Whole Earth Store.
- I'll see if I can find some vegetable juices that I really like (maybe I'll try fresh carrot juice).

- I'll start a small vegetable garden — just to see what it is like to grow my own lettuce, peas, etc.
- I'll spend less time at the local hangout — the temptation to "pig out" on junk food is too much to resist at that place.

Make a list of the obstacles and barriers to change. What are the kinds of things that stand in your way, that will make it hard to experiment with new food choices despite a conscious commitment to your nutritional well-being? How are you to make the adjustments and temporary sacrifices for longer term payoffs? Note a few obstacles on the same page of the log where you have listed one-month commitments. After each obstacle, list at least one plausible counterpoint. Be aware of the initial difficulties of making food changes.

Do you have trips planned that will complicate efforts to change? What about the influences of family and friends? How about the work environment, or the hassles you might encounter at school if you act differently from everybody else? What about myths?

Do you believe any of the following food-related myths: obesity is caused by heredity; it is "normal" to gain weight as you get older; fat runs in the family; exercise increases appetite; a slow metabolism cannot be changed; diet pills work; giving up junk food is not worth the effort; I'll inevitably gain weight if I stop smoking; and so on. All myths are true only if you believe in them.

Try not to be ambitious during the first month. You want early successes for confidence building — not awesome, energy-draining challenges that could rattle your confidence in your power to explore nutritious options. If you can find a friend to work with who has similar motivations (and his or her own log), so much the better.

Write a contract with yourself to carry out your plan. A written statement, appended to your food log, helps to build commitment by forming a clearer picture in your mind of what you are attempting and your resolve in going about it. State what you have decided to do in specific terms. You might want to post the self-contract in an obvious place where you will see it often. You can add visualizations to this step if you want an added push — develop images of your body growing more beautiful, stronger, younger looking, powerful, and admired.

Create a supportive environment for nutritional awareness. Design your physical environment so that it supports you in efforts to make wellness-centered food choices. Insure that your emotional and mental states are also consistent with the equilibrium and balance being fashioned in the nutritional dimension. This means that you should be continuing to pursue a balanced lifestyle as well as change in this one area. In the physical sense, you can shape a supportive environment by not having foods available which you are trying to eliminate, and by having in convenient places lots of desired munchies, such as varied fresh fruits and mixed bowls of raisins, cauliflower, radishes, celery, carrots, and so forth. Create a mood that fosters quiet, reflective dining and makes the occasion a beautiful celebration of friendship, life, health, or whatever you wish to make of it. For example, be conscious of the room lighting; burn incense; play music by Vivaldi or Mozart; place a vase of flowers on the table; light candles; think positive thoughts; and do whatever else along these lines appeals to you and affects the mood you want to fashion.

Become aware of negative nutritional norms. Look closely at what happens when you are with different kinds of groups that tend to make it more difficult, uncomfortable, and less enjoyable to choose food with deliberation and a focus on nutritional value rather than on hunger appeasement and entertainment. How much do you change these norms, or position yourself outside of their influence? You can become adept at doing both.

Step one is to pay attention to what is happening in the

cultures around you that affect your food preferences and choices. Avoid the company of junk-food junkies, and do those things that help you to feel good about yourself and that give you pleasure and positive self-esteem. The happier you are with you, the better your chances for treating yourself well in a nutritional sense.

Initiate a reading program. Go to the local library or bookstore and select a few publications on nutrition that look interesting to you (consider the Honor Roll recommendations). Peruse the books, knowing that you do not have to follow, believe, comprehend, or agree with all or any of the points being advocated. What ideas do you find most attractive and consistent with your own beliefs? What feelings do various nutritionists and others bring up for you? What interesting new concepts do you discover that you might want to implement? Make learning about this dimension an adventure instead of a dreary complexity. The key is your willingness to be casual and not intense or dogmatic, as are so many experts in this field. Naturally, you do not have to limit yourself to books or other written materials; if you have access to films, lectures, courses, or other forms of information about the subject, all the better. Whatever you like that appeals and attracts your curiosity is desirable.

Be generous in the use of self-rewards. When you try new patterns and find satisfaction in doing so, be good to yourself. Celebrate! Acknowledge yourself for having the commitment to make changes. Relish the slimmer, more energized you. Positive reinforcement is healthy and a sound force for increased motivation; negative reinforcement, such as self-criticism, put-downs, and guilt rarely do anyone any good.

Evaluate and make adjustments. At the end of the first plan period, evaluate how things have gone. Have the payoffs been worth the effort? What has been most difficult? What have been the major successes? The most important part of the process could take place at this time. Are you willing to revise your plan, reshape the contract, and make other adjustments in the process? The next time through should be a lot easier, and the payoffs at the end should be even better. Reflect, at least, on the experience of deliberate approaches to nutritional well-being. Consider additional ways to make conscious and informed food choices a part of your wellness lifestyle.

Try alternatives to food. Seriously, there are frequent instances when eating is done as a substitute for meeting other kinds of needs. Maybe you would gain more satisfaction (and less weight) from getting noticed or hugged.

Supplement your sources of information about food. One of the best sources of independent information is the Nutrition Action Project sponsored by the Center for Science in the Public Interest. This non-profit, tax-exempt watchdog organization monitors the food industry and its products, sponsors research, and produces consumer-oriented pamphlets, posters, and books. If you share my inclinations toward fresh vegetables, whole grains, beans, nonfat milk, fat reduction, cutbacks in salt, sugar, and other nonnutritive foods, you may enjoy the Project's monthly reports.*

Avoid taking the USDA's basic four food groups too seriously. What started out as a useful device for organizing a large body of information into an easily understandable system is now misused by such special interest groups as the National Dairy Council (NDC). The result is that a focus on the four food groups can do more harm than good. Among the major problems with the system are the following concerns:

· It can be used as a cover-up of our major nutritional difficulties. High blood cholesterol is linked in most studies with excessive sodium and saturated fat/cholesterol consumption. The four-food-group system ignores these is-

---

*Subscriptions cost $15 for one year — write CSPI Nutrition Action Project, 1755 S. Street NW, Washington, D.C., 20009.

sues, focusing only on vitamin, mineral, and protein values.

· It emphasizes groups of food rather than individual foods. The system does not identify a major reality of the standard U.S. diet, namely, that we eat too much highly processed, sugar-laden, and devitalized materials (I hesitate to use the word "foods"). You have no way of knowing, for example, that a typical breakfast cereal, "fortified with eight essential vitamins and minerals," derives more than 70 percent of its total calories from sugar and fat. A system that obscures this kind of specific information does not work.

· It is subject to abuse by special pleaders. Ice cream and chocolate pudding are touted by the NDC as examples of foods in the healthful milk group. The NDC also promotes egg yolks and butter as good sources of vitamin A (without, naturally, reminding us that our diet is already "saturated" with fat, sugar, and cholesterol). The average consumer probably does not realize that it would take *nine* eggs or a quarter-pound of butter to supply even a child's RDA for vitamin A.

In short, obtaining the RDA minimums is far less a problem than avoiding excesses of fat, sugar, additives, and salt. Displays in museums, hospitals, and other public places which purport to offer helpful nutritional information, when organized by food companies with products to sell, are automatically suspect. Know that the presence of individual vitamins and minerals is only a part of the nutritional adequacy picture; what a food does *not* have can be even more significant to your health than what it does.

Pull out all stops to raise your self-esteem. Ghastly food patterns, as with the lack of rigorous daily exercise, the absence of stress-management skills, unawareness of cultural reinforcements for worseness, and the failure to take personal responsibility for health, often can be traced to a poor self-concept or low self-esteem. Attempting to institute new food-selection and eating habits without an awareness of how food abuses serve as substitutes for other unmet needs will, in the long term, prove unsuccessful. To make significant advances in this and any other wellness dimension, you need something far more profound than technical detail about a scientific issue. Food is just one kind of nourishment; you also nourish yourself with caring relationships, good thoughts, and the like. Work at finding a peace within yourself. Know and value who you are and what you want to become, and be able to celebrate yourself for having the wisdom and courage to consciously pursue your best prospects. You are the only one who can decide what the height of those prospects can be — and this decision is vastly affected by your level of self-worth. Upgrading that is a no-lose proposition.

Enough! Time to move on, though the subject of eating for performance as well as enjoyment and good health has only been scratched. Do try to spend more time motivating yourself to eat for health enhancement rather than for the other five styles. Most importantly, go quietly and slowly but with confidence in your quest for your special ways to wellness dining.

Today's story reflects the idea, emphasized throughout this section, that you do not have to have all the answers all the time. A novitiate asked the Zen master, "What is death?"

"I do not know," said the master. Shocked, the student replied, "But you are the Zen master."

"Yes," he replied, "but I am not a dead Zen master."

With a fully alive and triumphant stroke, mark Day Eight complete.

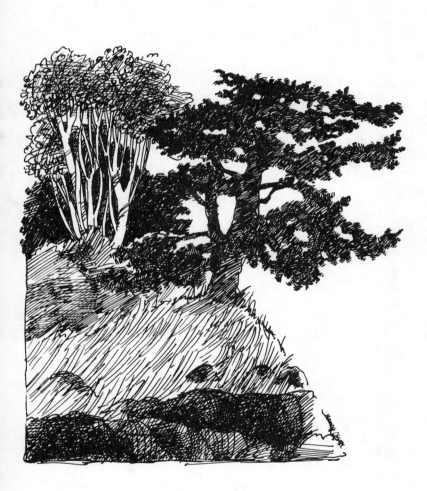

Day Nine

Understand The Dynamics Of Stress And Consider The Payoffs Of Stress Management

Purpose: In 15 minutes or so, you should have a thorough appreciation for the positive side of the stress dimension. Your purposes today are twofold: (1) to learn the simple basics of a topic that is misrepresented and unnecessarily made to seem complex and technical; and (2) to read about and ponder a few simple but effective strategies for minimizing the hazards and maximizing the benefits of the stress phenomenon.

The word "stress" has negative connotations in our society. It implies the presence of a standardized, unvarying, and uncontrollable outside force acting on your mind and body to create pressures and strains which can run you down and lead to nasty illnesses and an untimely demise. Surprise! This is only half-true, or more accurately, it is but one of two ways to think of and respond to stress. You have a choice.

Stress is also available as a source of energy. Stress can be seen as varied forms of opportunities, as events and circumstances subject to internal controls. Stress, in short, can be a positive and beneficial element, a steady fountain of motivation and creativity. It all depends on just two things: (1) your knowledge of the dynamics of stress; and (2) your ability to manage the stuff! Today you will learn about the dynamics of stress management; tomorrow and the next day you will become familiar with stress-management skills. (The day after and beyond, you can conquer the world — well, at least come to terms with it.)

THE DYNAMICS OF STRESS

A lot of books have been written about stress. Most of them are pretty good and all the authors have vast amounts of knowledge, experience, and techniques to convey. It never hurts to learn about such a vital dimension of wellness. At the back of this book, I critique and recommend a number of such works which are among my favorites. But you do not have to become an expert to know what is truly significant about stress; you do not have to read anything else if you do not wish to do so. You do want to develop a sense for: the physiology and sources of stress, the *positive* side of the phenomenon; the relationship of your performance in other wellness dimensions (e.g., fitness) with how successfully you deal with stress; your current effective or ineffective methods for dealing with stress; the variety of your interpretations and the power of "multiple-micros" versus overrated "occasional-macros" (I just made up these terms, but they are useful); and the preeminence of practice over knowledge. That was a long sentence; it may sound complicated. It is not. Remember, I am asserting that you can learn what is genuinely worth knowing about stress in 15 minutes (today) and can start to lock in these talents with a couple 15-minute practice sessions (Days Ten and Eleven).

Let's briefly examine each of the six aspects of the dynamics of stress, which I have just indicated are the basic insights you need to master this wellness dimension.

The Physiology and Sources of Stress

This could get complicated, and usually does with definitions, buzz words, and chemical jargon. There's nothing really wrong with this; it can be fascinating, in fact — but it can also be overdone, leading people to tune out and pay no attention.

People vary a great deal in the way they respond to the same events and circumstances. What is an energy-draining stress situation for one person can be an invigorating high for another. Why? Because, for varied reasons, some people learn to *interpret* things in a positive way — which is to say they *choose* to view things from an advantageous rather than a negative perspective. I'll give you an example. Suppose I laid a 4' x 12' board across your hot tub (or bathtub, bedpan, or whatever) and asked if you had the chutzpah to walk across it. No problem, right? You would no doubt waltz across. However, suppose I placed the same board between two eight-story buildings. Now if I asked, you would at least pause, and you might decline to "walk the plank." So, whether an event is stressful or not is relative or depends on your interpretation of the situation, your preparation, and so forth. Incidentally, I gave this example in a talk recently, and a large woman in the front row said, "No way, man! No way would I walk across that board if it were between tall buildings. You crazy or something?"

Thinking I would be extra clever, I asked, "But what if your child were in the other building, and it was on fire?"

She paused for a moment, then said, "Which child?" — which goes to show that one's stress level is based on how one interprets any event.

Stress is usually defined as a generalized response of the body to any demand. This means that the brain picks up some stimuli, decodes them, and thereby sets off a complex chain reaction. They key event in this process is the way in which the mind interprets, responds or adapts to the stimuli — no matter what the source of those stimuli. In real life terms, here is a partial account of what goes on in your body in response to stress: increased heart rate, metabolism, blood pressure and flow, lactate levels, a-drenalin and noradrenalin reactions, and constricted blood vessels. There's more, but this gives you the idea of the stress response.

The average person experiences 1,042 stress events every day,* all of which derive from three basic sources: environmental, physical, and mental. Environmental sources include the weather, sounds, and the like. Physical stresses are similar but organic — animals, crowds, and individuals. These two sources are important, but less pervasive than the third variety — the mental stresses. This source is composed of all the other things that trigger the physiological reactions just mentioned. It includes everything that you *choose* to get worked up about, including time pressures, frustrations, glorious achievements, and so forth. Thus, you can readily appreciate that there are at least 1,042 daily opportunities to get stressed — *if* you do not take charge of things.

The reality of stress and the importance of doing something constructive about it are not contemporary discoveries. A physician named Edmund Jacobson published a book about this wellness dimension in 1929 (*Progressive Relaxation*), based on his laboratory work at Harvard beginning in 1908. If there is any change in the way things are now, it is probably only in the increased extent of stress in modern life — and a far greater prevalence of harmful ways for poorly informed Americans to deal with it (i.e., excessive reliance upon healers and medicines).

---

*While this sounds impressive and authoritative, the truth is I made it up. There is no such creature as an average person.

The Positive Face Of Stress

Stress is usually presented as a silent but pervasive hazard. It is usually considered a major factor if not the primary cause of dozens of gruesome diseases and disabilities. In fact, there is a debate in some circles as to whether it is the major factor in heart disease or cancer. Furthermore, there are debates as to which professions and occupations suffer the most from it — air traffic controllers, policemen, accountants (during the tax-preparation season), athletes, and so forth. There are, I suspect, some latent status considerations in all this — "My job is pretty deadly, but I'm toughing it out," or "Anyone would act crazy who has to do what I do."

So, the second dynamic to remember about stress is that it does not *have* to be seen from the negative point of view. Be suspicious of interpretations that confuse a basic, essential demand upon your body as inevitably leading to unpleasant reactions and outcomes. It all depends on what you say to yourself about the everyday events and circumstances to which you are exposed. Decide that you will reserve the right — and the power — to interpret all stimuli in a way that best serves your conscious purposes. In doing so, you will quickly realize that stress is definitely not synonymous with distress, that choices are available, and that the positive facet of this stress phenomenon is ever so much more attractive and useful than the prevailing negative connotation.

The Interconnectedness of Wellness Dimensions

Stress awareness and management is a vital, irreplaceable skill for anyone committed to the pursuit of his/her highest potentials for whole-person excellence. As you will sense from the materials in Days Nine through Eleven, this dimension by itself provides splendid capabilities for personal effectiveness. However, a third consideration about the dynamics of stress, which I think will serve you, is that an awareness and practice of stress management is not optimal. It may be sufficient for most people, and a capability in this dimension would certainly represent an advance in terms of population health levels, but for your goal of high-level wellness, there is more. Appreciate the fact that your performance in one area (in this case, ability to manage and utilize stress energies) is affected by your consciousness and participation in the other four wellness dimensions. For example, the capability of your body to adapt and respond, to withstand and endure, to process and interpret enormous quantities of sensations and other stimuli is very much affected by your level of physical conditioning and daily energy expenditures, your nutrient levels, grounding and sense of emotional and spiritual well-being, and similar balances and strengths. Without attention to a balanced lifestyle, the utilization of deep breathing, visualization, and other stress-management skills could degenerate into palliative gimmickry. In this case, an isolated relaxation technique could become a hollow and useless symptom suppressor, as dysfunctional a "magic bullet" as the quick fix (i.e., the pill) it should supplant. So, keep in mind that, however useful this and the other dimensions are, each is a part of a larger whole.

Becoming Aware of Current Responses

You *already have* a vast repertoire of mechanisms, techniques, and patterns for dealing with the great range and quantity of ordinary stresses, as well as the occasional zingers (e.g., job loss, rejection by a friend, etc.). The problem is, you probably are not aware of most of them, many work only part of the time, and almost none are consciously practiced to channel stresses toward optimal returns. Furthermore, some of the responses you learned over the years (subconsciously) are less than effective; they actually make matters worse by creating other problems (e.g., smoking, kicking the dog, munching out, popping pills, and so on).

Most Americans have learned a method of stress management from television commercials. The method is called "pill popping." The solution to nervous indigestion, tension headaches, alcohol-induced hangovers, sleepless nights and a score of "media maladies" is the magic bullet (tranquilizer) available at the drugstore. While some doctors are insisting that as much as 70 percent of all suffering derives from boredom, unhappiness, anxiety, and purposelessness, many continue to treat people as though their basic problem is a Valium deficiency.

There are several complications in this approach to stress management. One is that it does not work; another is that it sometimes leads to serious side effects; and a third is that it does nothing to help the individual cope with underlying lifestyle problems, which are likely to become more rather than less severe.

Therefore, one of the early "action" steps you will be taking is to inventory your stress-response patterns to discover what works and what does not. You might be surprised to learn that your methods and techniques are vastly influenced by parents and other role models, and that so little is chosen in a conscious manner. More important, you will almost certainly enjoy the process of assessing the range of choices available to you and the satisfying returns attendant upon a disciplined and aware stress-management capability.

Individual Responses to Stress and the Power of "Little Things"

A popular idea in the literature about stress is that there is a limit to the amount of change, crises, or major events which we can handle in a given time period without falling ill, or worse. This, at any rate, is the thesis of Dr. Thomas Holmes, who developed and popularized the "Life Change Index." The Index contains 43 life-change situations, each of which is assigned a certain point value. According to Dr. Holmes, the more points you accumulate within a year, the more likely you are to get sick.

This concept is useful and helpful in demonstrating that stresses are cumulative. Beyond that, it has shortcomings. It implies that we are equally affected by given experiences. The death of a spouse, for example, has an item value of 100 points, a jail term (not specific about the length!) is 63 points, a mortgage over $10,000 (does *anybody* have a mortgage for less?) is 31 points, and Christmas is 12 points. Personally, I think the implication that values (points) can be generalized to apply equally for everybody is silly. Marital separation (65 points) could be upsetting to the degree stated for some, but would be a welcome and liberating blessing without any negative effects for others. So, one big problem with the scale is that it does not account for our uniqueness, for the fact that how we interpret a given stress event is more consequential than the event itself. It is our reaction to events, in other words, which determines whether we suffer or prosper as a consequence of what happens to us.

The other problem is that the major impact of stress, for better or worse, is not revealed in our experience of or reaction to 43 life-change events, as the Holmes scale suggests. These big developments, which I term "occasional macro" events, happen infrequently in our lives. I mean, how many times a week — or even a year — does your spouse die (100 points)? How often did you go to jail last month (63 points)? Retired lately (45 points)? You get the picture. In my opinion, based on observations at wellness centers across the country and on interviews with hundreds of people who are working on their own specialized approaches to optimal functioning, the "occasional macros" are not the key issues in dealing effectively with the dimension of stress. The genuine challenge is to manage the hundreds of items, or little life events and circumstances, that come up every day.

These are the issues which test your stress awareness and management capabilities. Nothing glamorous or fearsome about these little challenges and hazards — they include a ringing alarm, burned toast, heavy rain or deep cold, a flat tire or dead battery, a crowded freeway or stalled bus, confusion about a work task, conflicts between appointments, ringing phones, a headache, missed exercise, and so on, day after day. We all have our own lists, and the lists change somewhat every day. By themselves, these "multiple micros" do not seem like much, but they accumulate and result in effects far more pervasive than the dramatic cave-ins of roofs, holocausts, and other perditions and acts-of-God which can ruin your day (the "occasional macros"). So, start to pay attention to these little things because little things mean a lot.

I'm fond of a poem called "The Broken Shoelace" by Charles Bukowski which makes the point in another way :

It's not the large things in life that drive a man to the madhouse.
It's not the death of his love
But a shoelace that breaks with no time left.

The Limited Utility of Isolated Knowledge

In order to develop a capacity to respond effectively to stress-producing events and circumstances, a certain information base about this wellness dimension is essential. The principles for stress management, techniques for relaxation and centering, and ideas for channeling stress energies for productivity, are invaluable. Such knowledge represents the foundation for one of the vital skill areas of a wellness lifestyle. Unfortunately, knowledge without practice is of almost no use. It is true that you can engage in informative discussions with others (and elicit the B.F. Hutton syndrome) as you describe the dynamics of the stress phenomenon, but you cannot "cash in" on this talent unless you use it. This simply means that you must put some time aside when you have completed the knowledge-gathering phase of this book to try out the concepts, experiment with the exercises, and adopt or modify the approaches to your own individual style and pattern. Then, put it all to work in the context of your personal wellness plan. You will thereby increase your chances for maximum personal effectiveness while avoiding the frustrations of "knowing better" but being stuck in distressful complacency.

To summarize the knowledge component (practice time is coming up), recall that the body and mind work in interconnected ways. Stress comes from many physical, environmental and mental sources, and the physiological effects of all varieties of stress are predictable. How you *choose* to respond to stress is of greater significance than the events or circumstances, and it makes great sense to think more about the positive effects of stress than about the hazards or negative consequences of poor stress adaptation. It is important to maintain a balanced wellness lifestyle as part of your stress-management repertoire, and vital to develop a conscious awareness of how you already deal with specific stresses. In this way, you are able to make adjustments in the interest of added personal effectiveness, and to better manage the large number of relatively minor aggravations, demands, and pressures. The cumulative effects of these forces, though individually trivial, are more consequential than the impact of the relatively rare major events on your ability to stay balanced, maintain your equilibrium, and safeguard your degree of control.

Finally, as just noted, knowledge is wisdom when it is linked with practice and use, and the satisfactory experience of desired results. Consider the following sentiments expressed by Duane Grimstad, the chaplain of the St. Helena Health and Hospital Center:

> Have you ever stood on the windy shore of the Pacific and watched the Monterey Pines as they are bowed and twisted, up and down, back and forth by the prevailing winds? Even the great Pacific storms

cannot unearth these trees. Each gust and gale seems to strengthen their resolve to remain where they have grown....

How can they take it — that buffeting day and night forever? The answer is simple: Deep roots that cling to subterranean rocks and soil, roots that are shaped to grip unrelentingly, roots that never let go, roots that don't know the meaning of retreat, roots on the windward side....

This "root growing" doesn't happen overnight. It is a process over a period of years that produces strong roots to defy the storms....

What conclusion can we draw from these thoughts? Welcome the little winds of trial and disappointment. They build character. Then, when the storms of life come, we can take the beating like the sturdy Pines of Monterey for we have roots on the windward side.

THE MANAGEMENT OF STRESS

The objective of stress management as part of a wellness lifestyle is to channel stress energies for productive results. In this approach, the basic goal is to *achieve* desired satisfactions and payoffs; an important *side effect* is that dangerous hazards and illnesses associated with stress build-up are *minimized* or avoided altogether. This, of course, is a departure from the usual emphasis on coping with adversity and minimizing problems as the primary goal.

The wellness approach to stress management, as with nutrition and fitness, is that the best defense against the negatives is a strong offense aimed at achieving the positives. In this approach, good results automatically prevent bad effects.

The first component of this positive orientation to stress management is awareness. This means that you develop a sensitivity to how your mind and body subconsciously interpret and initially signal a perception of stress events and circumstances, and that you develop a self-programmed readiness to direct these inner cues and hints into productive responses. You are already on your way to developing this awareness with the knowledge you now have about the dynamics of stress. In Days Ten and Eleven, you will be learning a few enjoyable methods, such as deep breathing and visualization, for channeling and managing stress. In the minutes remaining today, just consider a few strategies consistent with the above dynamics that should further strengthen your management capabilities.

USEFUL STRATEGIES FOR STRESS MANAGEMENT

The following list is but a sample of attitudes and activities that logically follow from what has been noted about constructive approaches to stress management. I have found these to be useful, but there are hundreds of other interesting strategies noted in the various books written about this dimension, including those recommended in the "Honor Roll" at the back of this book. Consider this list, take a look at a few other sets of stress-management ideas, and then write your own observations as you go along, testing and refining all the while. Before you know it, you will be an expert.

Distinguish momentary feelings from unchangeable facts. Your first reaction to a stressful event — based on years of "normal" and customary programming — may be to get depressed, to panic, to worry, or to become very angry. Under certain circumstances, any of these feelings may be appropriate in helping to get the results that serve you. Most of the time, however, these feelings are *not* appropriate, as they divert you from experiencing optimal returns and rising above the "absence of illness" stage of the Worseness/Wellness Continuum. Whether appropriate or not at the moment, it is never in your interest, from a stress-management or other wellness orientation, to stay in a frump, huff, or similar "discombobbled" place. You can choose not to. Remind yourself now — before you become upset — to recall that the choice to move on to other feelings can and should be made. Pay attention to upsets when you habitually interpret something that way. Then, think about other feelings and moods available, and start consciously reprogramming yourself accordingly.

Expect stresses, plan for them, and thereby make them less upsetting. You cannot go around "blissed out" all the time. You would not want to if you could. As Jay Cleve suggests, a time without stress would be like going to a party and spending the evening in the closet with the coats — not stressful, to be sure, just a secure experience. A person in a continual state of deep relaxation is not a potent force in the world. Take a pencil and paper, and a look at your watch. Give yourself just three minutes for a little exercise. Make a list of everyday events and circumstances which usually bring on some degree of stress response. Try not to censor yourself.

Finished? Fine. Now look at your list. *Take responsibility for the presence of those stresses!* Do this by examining the "payoffs" you derive by allowing these conditions to persist, day after day. If you can see the "gains" you obtain from even negative situations, the negative look of the situation is lightened. For example, you may have noted "time pressures," or something related to the fact that there is too much to do in too little time. Join the crowd. Most people feel that way, a lot if not all the time. It is usually due to attempting too much. This is the point. By recognizing that certain stresses are necessary and normal in the course of getting or doing something you value, and by consciously expecting the stresses, you naturally and effortlessly become less taxed by these conditions. "Anticipate and mitigate" might be a useful rule in this case.

Work on your stress-management vital signs. Unfortunately, the stress dimension's equivalent for the exercise physiologist's maximum oxygen uptake (VO^2) and recovery heart rate have not been scientifically or technically proven. Do not let that stand in your way; go ahead and develop your own subjective indicators of where you are now in order to chart improvements as you go along. For instance, make note of how you reacted to given stresses before you started to develop an awareness of the dynamics of stress management. Perhaps you would want to write a brief summary of how things used to be in a diary or log of some kind. Note how you once took things so seriously and heavily, how you would jump off bridges at the least upset, how you perceived every slight and disappointment as the beginning of the end, and so on. As your stress-management skills are practiced and satisfactions are derived from your successes, you will find delight in observing how much power and control you have relative to where you were when the program started. That, of course, is the highest purpose of wellness vital signs, even if they are not objectively measurable. You know it works, and that is what counts.

Learn how to break your body's stress code. At first, it may seem mysterious and secretive, but you can learn to recognize what stress looks and feels like. There is a wide-ranging list of symptoms which are associated with a build-up of negative physiological conditions. If you become alert to these signals, you will know when to practice a chosen technique to regain optimal mind/body balance. In general, distress-code symptoms are muscle tightness (including twitches and tremors), neck- and backaches, stiff shoulders, stomach "knots" and irritations, constipation, headaches, grinding teeth, dry mouth, nervous irritability, foot or hand tapping, smoking, sweaty palms or brows and, of course, zits.

Fortunately, awareness makes all the difference. Knowing the code is a necessary first step in reducing negative stress and increasing enjoyment of life. So, pay attention to how you carry stress, what your body does as stress builds up, and how you react to it. You only make things worse by trying to ignore what your body and mind are trying to tell you. In itself, this awareness will not solve problems, but it will help you comprehend the reality of physical distress and get serious about doing something constructive to avoid or mitigate it.

Pursue excellence in the other wellness dimensions. I have mentioned it before, but the theme bears sounding again. You will derive stress-management benefits from initiatives in every one of the other four wellness dimensions. That is why the wellness concept is such an effective complement to a truly good and full life. By integrating the key dimensions, you realize a multiplier or synergistic effect beyond the sum of the different investments. This is especially noticeable in the case of physical fitness. A commentary in the *Journal of the American Medical Association* (Aug. 3, 1979, 242, 5, pp. 427-28) discussed the scientific basis for the so-called "runner's high" and other forms of (pleasant) "altered states" attendant upon extreme exertion. It seems that brain hormones called endorphins play a major role in altering mood, emotion, and behavior. While the exact processes by which these beneficial effects are induced are not completely understood, their relationship to the maintenance of homeostasis is acknowledged. By practicing aerobic exercise every day, by eating nutritious and satisfying meals in a quiet and thoughtful way, by accepting responsibility for your feelings at all times, and by designing supportive environments, you can create a shield around your life that blocks out most of the discordant events and circumstances. Furthermore, what gets through is more easily within your power to manage and channel, given the capacity and preparedness you will have developed after Days Ten and Eleven.

Become an expert in stress resolution. "Resolving" a stressful event or circumstance does not always mean "solving" the situation. Many times, there *is* no perfect answer, or even a reasonably agreeable one. It is, in short, not always (often) possible to come up with a Solomon-like conclusion that pleases all parties. Therefore, your special challenge is to deal with the event or circumstance in a manner that seems best to you, and then move on to other matters! Frustration and indecision are hazardous to your health and your freedom to pursue wellness. A poor or mediocre decision is far better for your overall well-being than the demanding and debilitating stress effects of unresolved tensions while you search in vain for a terrific decision.

Work on developing a positive outlook on events and circumstances you cannot or do not wish to change. Anthony Raubitschek, Professor Emeritus of Classics at Stanford University (and recent recipient of the university's highest award for excellence in teaching, whose packed lectures earn standing ovations), was queried as to what he does for relaxation. "Relaxation?" he asked. "The best way to relax is to do two or three things at the same time. At the moment I am rereading Plato, the New Testament, and some Demosthenes" (*The Stanford Observer*, March 1979, p. 2).

Here are a couple of examples illustrating the simple process of changing your viewpoint about something and finding a diversion, from the lives of two friends named Frances Atkinson and Peter Allen. First, Frances:

It was a Sunday afternoon in July, and I was returning from Denver to the mountain cabin I had rented for the summer. As always, I could hardly wait to get back to my beautiful private retreat. Situated several miles above Evergreen, "my" cabin nestled among pines, aspen, and columbine in the heart of the big meadow country. Mt. Evans and other above-timberline peaks circle the horizon, and the silence is like a healing balm.

That Sunday, I started up Bear Creek Canyon, the

route I had chosen because I love its scenery. But I had forgotten that I might find myself behind a slow driver; the Canyon highway isn't a four- or six-lane speedway like I-70. And sure enough — there I was in a slow line of traffic. Five cars ahead loomed the culprit. He drove a long black Oldsmobile with a passenger in the seat beside him and three more in the back seat. I don't know how impatient the four drivers between us were, but *I* was mighty annoyed. Taking out my frustrations on other drivers (who can't hear me) is one of my hobbies, so I began:

"Good grief, Charley Brown! Is that all the faster you can manage in that overgrown limousine? This road isn't *that* tricky! You'll make it even if you do step it up to 20. C'mon!"

Every now and then he acted as though he'd heard me; he'd go five miles an hour faster for a little way, and then back we'd all lapse to 25 mph. I looked at my watch. I'm behind schedule, I thought to myself. I wanted to be up the mountain by 4 o'clock, and I'll never make it.

"Darnit, Buster — put your foot on that gas pedal and let's go! Can't you drive?" There was no chance of passing him. Some drivers . . . !

Suddenly I noticed we were rounding the curve of one of my favorite beauty spots: a winding quarter of a mile where the clear waters of Bear Creek rush and tumble over sharp rocks, and red, wooded cliffs rise high behind and above the sparkling creek. "How gorgeous!" I said aloud. And I began to let the gratitude-attitude take over. As I did so, I felt my body relax. How incredibly tense I'd been! My solo ranting against the driver up ahead had done nothing to him — only to me. My stomach had been tight, my fingers had been clenched around the steering-wheel, and my shoulders had been practically grabbing my neck and throat. What a relief, to let go of anger! And I laughed out loud.

Enjoy the trip, I told myself. I hardly needed reminding at that point that I had been missing the fantastic beauty around me, only because of my own frame of mind. Nobody else had taken that enjoyment away from me — only *I* had. And in the process, my body had paid a price, and so had my emotions — to say nothing of the fact that I had ignored the ever-present God-power which brought forth all of the beauty around me in the first place.

It felt good to be back to the nitty-gritty. What difference did it *really* make what time I got to my cabin? It would still be there. Certainly, arriving in one piece was more important than watching the clock. But most essential of all was my enjoying every square inch of and every second of that trip up the mountain. *This* was wellness: living each moment and experience to the hilt, with full mind-awareness, spirit-awareness; letting oneself be washed and cleansed by the pure stream of thankfulness and appreciation. And allowing one's cup to be filled, as in the words of the ancient sage, "Full measure, pressed down and running over!"

The black Oldsmobile led us up the canyon all the way to Evergreen. When the driver turned off the main road to his destination, I wished that I were close enough to thank him for making me drive slowly through all the beauty. For it was true that after I quieted down inside, the afternoon turned out to be one of the loveliest I've ever had. I spotted secluded places and discovered unusual rock formations I'd never seen before — all because I wasn't hurrying.

Just yesterday I was tempted to be impatient behind the wheel again. But I thought of my unknown friend who slowed me down, and I quickly shifted my mental and emotional gears from "hurry-itis" to "enjoy-itis." Automatically, my body relaxed. My route at that moment was along Speer Boulevard and 11th Avenue, and suddenly I found that the tall trees along Cherry Creek were dressed in lovely fall colors, and there were shrubs and tiny trees I'd never noticed before. What fun! And, I thought, who cares if this traffic causes me to miss the next three lights? From now on, I'm going to enjoy the trip!*

Peter likes to sketch when stressed by the pressure of exams. When he sent the following examples of his relaxation method to me, Peter wrote:

> *Art is one of my best approaches for dealing with problems. It helps me feel less fragmented; I flow between myself as the artist and the world I am drawing. Students in college like myself lack meaningful relaxation outlets to vent scholastic and other, existential, problems and doubts. Drawing, painting, sculpting, yoga, and running are my pressure reducers.*

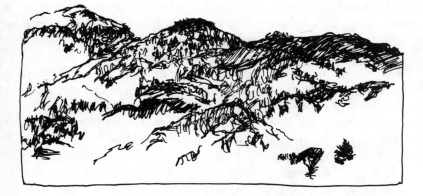

---

*Frances Atkinson, *Colorado Holistic Health Newsletter*, (Nov. 1978), pp. 2-3.

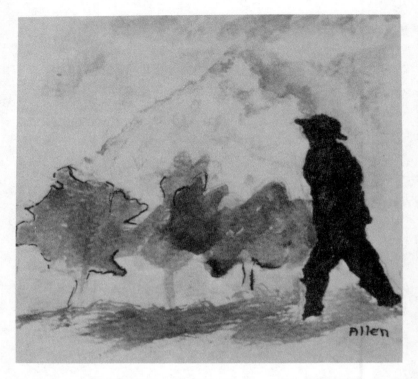

Inventory the "demand load" of your cultures. Be alert to overt and subtle ways that your job, family, and friendship cultures place stress upon you. Do those in authority lay excessive expectations or responsibilities on your desk? Is it considered not OK to ask for help? Is it expected that you will do "anything" for parents and relatives, even to the neglect of your own needs? Is there an unwritten "law" that the people who get promoted are those who behave like accountants at tax time — all year round? Look again at those things you listed as events and circumstances causing you stress. How many of these factors are, in reality, stresses that you once thought were a "normal" part of life because everybody else in your group or organization seemed to be experiencing them? More important, now that you recognize the varied ways that your cultures lay stress on you, what are you willing to do to mitigate or avoid these unhealthy, and unnecessary, demands?

Be creative and do something outrageous on occasion. Use your imagination to act out. Tell somebody off, release steam, amuse yourself and take a few risks. For example, maybe you glance at the ingredients on the label of Country Time Lemonade (which is advertised as being just like Grandma made it), and you know she never could have concocted such a brew without an advanced degree in chemistry! Or, you bite into a spoonful of Quaker Oats "all natural" granola (trusting James Fixx because he wrote a popular running book and thus could not be all bad), only to discover that the product has 23% brown sugar (and there ain't nothing natural about that, boys and girls). All of a sudden, you're ticked off. Why not go to the nearest window and shout: "I'm mad as hell and I'm not going to take it anymore!" Such a routine, acted in the proper spirit, could make you feel better, release a bit of tension, and provide your neighbors (and you) with a good laugh.

Or, try a routine something like that of consumer champion and TV character Herb Denenberg of Pennsylvania (former University of Pennsylvania professor, state insurance commissioner, and U.S. Senate candidate), who wears a white sanitation worker-type jumpsuit and a large plastic trash can called "Denenberg's Dump" into which he ceremoniously "files" products that deserve to be there. Believing that "the public has been screwed long enough," Denenberg now makes a career getting righteously indignant (for the TV cameras) about consumer rip-offs. Denenberg is, however, selective about his choice of targets. Asked about the problem of rat feces in chocolate, he replied, "So what? Who cares? I can't get excited about that. How about all the artificial sweeteners and chemical poisons they get in chocolate? That's what we should be attacking. I mean, a little rat shit never hurt anybody." And a little temper tantrum won't hurt you, either, so long as you don't take yourself too seriously. Robin Williams, or "Mork" of ABC TV's "Mork and

Mindy" show, calls this process "staying bozo," which has value as a defense mechanism against "the harsher realities of life on earth" (*Time*, March 12, 1979, *113*, 11, p. 2). It could be good for your soul, every so often.

There are other useful strategies for stress management, of course. Unless you are an accomplished speed reader, however, you already must be more than 15 minutes into Day Nine. Please excuse — I do get carried away at times. The mention of speed reading brings to mind the story about Woody Allen taking such a course and thereafter reporting that he read Tolstoy's *War and Peace* in six minutes. Asked to discuss the plot, he reported that it concerned Russians and fighting. Speed is not everything.

Let me acknowledge a few aspects that deserve attention, such as time management. At some point, it might make a lot of sense to take a short course, read a book, or just examine an article on this subject. Organizing things a bit better at work and home gives you greater control. Good work habits and better all-around time utilization can help you focus, set priorities, and minimize wasted efforts.

Another area relevant to stress management is that of directionality. If you can generally arrange your activities so as to serve life purposes, you will be setting things up for stress to work for you. Naturally, this necessitates that you make time to reflect upon your current values, your goals for the year, and your fundamental purposes.

Yet another attitudinal technique is to "Betamax" yourself in order to go to the bank with your recent stress experiences. That is, profit from how you responded to a stressful event or circumstance by recalling your behaviors and feelings in the manner of a detached, uninvolved observer. Do not fault yourself or wish you had thought, done, or said something else. Just observe the transaction. In view of what you have learned about stress dynamics and management, what do you notice about your role in these recent experiences? Try this form of detached observation several times. It is an essential phase to the profitable next step of behavior rehearsal.

As the term implies, "behavior rehearsal" is knowing how you want to be (in this case, centered, grounded, and capable of using stress energies in a positive and useful manner), and practicing *being* that way. You can always predict that, based on past experience, certain stresses will arise again; rather than improvise when they do, prepare for these times. You can do this by running through, mentally and physically, how you choose to respond in light of new understanding and motivation regarding the management and channeling of stress energies.

Finally, a word or two must be given to music, faith, myths, rituals, retreats, good work, and mutual supports as mechanisms that have been employed throughout civilization. These are intuitive — people come upon them naturally, without effort or special training. Usually, these forms are not consciously appreciated for their stress-management purposes. The fact is, our ancestors employed these forms before we ever thought of fancy words and scientific explanations for dealing with upsets, challenges, and all the other myriad conditions and circumstances great and incidental to which the body/mind is heir. Nevertheless, they can and will work for us — and already do. The trick is to selectively develop, consciously apply, and more skillfully utilize these timeless measures for our own contemporary needs and ends.

This concludes Day Nine. Excuse if I got carried away — there is so much value in the dynamics and management of stress. If Day Nine required more than 15 minutes, well, *mea culpa.*

Make a bold mark at the back signaling another milestone in your advance toward getting hooked on wellness. Glad you are staying with it — thanks for participating.

Californians are pretty adept at stress management. They have to be in order to cope with rapid changes, what with all the cults, kooks, fads, and trends. One result is that relationships often do not last very long. It is not uncommon, when a couple is breaking up, for one of the mates to remark: "How could you do this to me, after I gave you the best hours of my week?"

Enjoy the rest of the day.

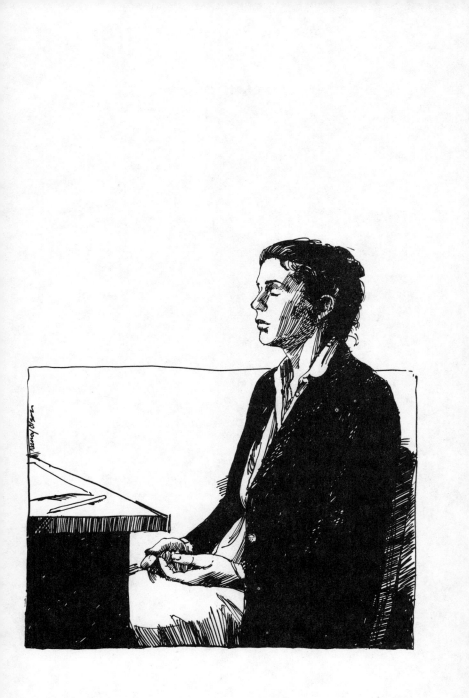

Day Ten

Learn And Practice Deep Breathing And Muscle Relaxation For Stress Management

Purpose: When you complete the reading for this day, you should be capable and willing to practice some form of a preparatory relaxation technique on a regular basis. In doing so, you will be able to reverse physical and psychological symptoms of excessive stress, and respond to it in optimal ways for added personal effectiveness.

Think of stress as a form of energy. This energy is neither good nor bad; as with electrical energy, it can illuminate, power and otherwise serve, or it can shock the pants off you. How you interpret and handle it makes all the difference — and the difference can be extraordinary. The difference, in short, is a choice between the efficient use or profligate waste of your resources. Or, wellness versus worseness.

So, to recap from Day Nine, remember that stress is an irreplaceable ingredient for getting aroused about life, and for keeping up your interest. Recall also that the effect of stress is dependent not on the events or circumstances which precipitate it, but rather how it is experienced. This, of course, depends upon you. You already have an awareness of stress dynamics and attitudes for effective coping. Now you can develop confidence in your capacity to consciously choose responses that are appropriate and consistent with nearly any situation, and be aware of the creative and adaptive options that serve your highest purposes. Such confidence is, in part, a function of your stress-management skills. Day Ten concentrates on two preliminary skills that are essential for personal effectiveness: the regular practice of deep breathing, and muscle relaxation.

DEEP BREATHING

There is a dramatic difference between breathing to sustain life and breathing to enhance well-being. While the former is preferable to not breathing at all, it leaves a lot to be desired. An attitude of breathing as not anything more than a necessary survival process is comparable to viewing health as the absence of illness. It will get you by at the margins, but will also entail more than your fair share of lost opportunities.

Deep breathing techniques are invaluable for wellness. They take a minimal amount of time and provide immediate payoffs. The payoffs are both physical and psychological when regularly employed for stress-awareness and management purposes.

You do not need a guru, a mantra, or an expensive course to utilize these techniques. You need not go to the mountain or sit cross-legged on a rock. And no, you do not have to wear strange costumes or stare at the sun. The deep breathing and other relaxation skills described in Days Ten and Eleven necessitate (1) a basic awareness that voluntary control of emotional states is possible; (2) a bit of experimentation and practice; and (3) the regular use of chosen forms.

Do emphasize the positive: the benefits really are better than the illnesses foregone. They include an increase in energy, improved concentration, better alertness to subtle signs and indicators, the restoration of an inner balance, and an ability to achieve, at will, a mood of external serenity. There are other advantages, but these alone seem sufficient reasons to give deep breathing a try.

Yoga practitioners view breathing as more than simple oxygen nourishment for cells and tissues, and more than a fuel for the production of vital bodily processes. To the yoga philosopher, the manner of breathing affects the quality of life force. Breathing affects and is affected by mood. Change the pace and flow of your breathing, and you regulate at will the feelings you experience. You need not be a yoga philosopher or practitioner to know that! The exercise suggestions coming up build on this awareness. Breathing must become a conscious process to effect deep relaxation.

Getting Started

There are probably hundreds of ways to set up a stress-management experience using breathing-relaxation exercises. The following exercise is just a sample; as in everything else, you are encouraged to play with variations and to try other ways, but this should help you get started. Read through the rest of this section, then go back and try the different steps.

· Choose a suitable location and time for a quiet minute or two. You need two kinds of refuge — one that you can slip into, sort of like Clark Kent's telephone booth, and one you can visit when you have a bit more time (like a beach, trail or park). Think of a few such spots.
· Get comfortable. Loosen or remove tight clothing, shoes, and jewelry.
· Take a deep breath. (You probably were wondering when I would finally get around to having you do it.)
· Take another deep breath. This time, inhale through your nose, exhale through your mouth. Take your sweet

time about it, allowing your abdomen to rise and descend fully and gently with this in-and-out cycle.
· Get rhythmic and slow with your relaxation breathing. The in-and-out cycles should be about equal in length. Go deeper than shallow, upper-chest breathing. Your chest should barely move, while your abdomen should expand and contract.
· Notice if you feel any tension in your neck, shoulder, lower back, or elsewhere. No need to do anything about it, yet. Just be aware of a tendency to carry tension in certain parts of your body.
· Glance at a timepiece and note the second-hand. Continue your rhythmic breathing as noted above, and count the number of full breaths you take in one minute. Unless you have obstructed lung function or are not breathing properly, you are probably taking four or fewer breath cycles in the space of a minute.
· Connect breathing with pleasant thoughts. Nothing spectacular for the moment, just pictures that create further comfort and calm. Try thinking of a deep pattern of blue; imagine the oxygen you inhale as soothing, and think of your body as warm and heavy.
· Make a sound as you exhale. Choose a steady, lengthy note, such as *humm*. Let the sound vibrate, massaging your abdomen, brain, and any other part to which you want to draw attention (e.g., a tense muscle).
· Consider that air drawn into your lungs is pure energy, and that exhaled air is spent gas (i.e., carbon dioxide waste products) that have served and are no longer needed.
· Practice these breathing exercises.
· Devise variations, using different positions (i.e., standing, sitting, lying down, hanging upside down, and so on).
· Do a few conscious breathing rituals at least three times a day, several minutes per session for the next three weeks. After that, do the breathing as you feel the need

— or more accurately, the opportunity to employ the technique.

MUSCLE RELAXATION

Some things do not become obvious until, for various reasons, we decide to pay attention. An approaching storm, for example, may not be evident until the thunder and lightning bolts appear. Some people, though, have trained themselves to detect subtle atmospheric changes long before the darkening sky. Similarly, your awareness of the time of day, the mood of a friend, or other situations varies in accord with the degree of perceptiveness you have been encouraged to develop regarding that situation. Regrettably, body awareness is not a skill emphasized in the home, school, or other environments of most people. Deep breathing habits are a first step in raised awareness of subtleties in physical states; the recognition of muscle patterns and progressive relaxation of specific muscle groups is a second step in this direction.

Muscle-relaxation exercises will help you become more aware of your inner processes and your deeper self. These activities will, in effect, quiet your spirit and lead to marked physical changes conducive to relaxation. Combined with deep breathing, the physical effects include diminished oxygen consumption, reduced heartbeat and blood pressure, and lower carbon dioxide and respiration rates. Further, muscle secretions of lactic acid (related to tension) and the frequency/intensity of brain-wave patterns also change into forms consistent with moods of serenity and calm.

In addition to these physical changes, muscle relaxation can be employed to ease the symptoms of various illnesses, to mitigate hostile or depressive tendencies, and to improve concentration.

Muscle relaxation compares very favorably with the use of pill popping. The former has no unpleasant side effects, does not cost a lot of money, is always available without a prescription, and gets getter results when used as directed.

Dr. Edmund Jacobson, mentioned yesterday as the author of *Progressive Relaxation*, is usually credited with starting the popular use of this technique. His theory was that we "store" tension, distress, or upset in various muscles. Unless we relieve this build-up, the body experiences fatigue and other problems related to an energy blockage in one or more burdened muscle groups. His exercises did just that: they allowed for the release of tension in a sequence, or progression, in a brief time period. All the writing and training by an assortment of experts ever since have been variations of Dr. Jacobson's muscle-relaxation techniques (including those noted below).

You may have chronically tense muscles and not be aware of the fact on a conscious level. Then again, you may not. Either way, you will enjoy and benefit from taking this next step in stress management. Muscle tension obstructs blood flow to tissues and cells, inhibits nutrient distribution throughout the body, and generates wastes and toxins. So, who needs it? It pays to pay attention, to become alert to such an important matter. Though a reality, you have to wonder: "How could something so powerful as muscle tension be overlooked by so many?" Who knows? The encouraging fact is that with a minimum of practice, progressive muscle relaxation will become quite natural, effective, and effortless.

With all this said, the time has come to get on with it.

Getting Started

As with the preparatory steps in deep breathing, muscle-relaxation exercises should be facilitated by the choice and design of supportive environments and positions. Make sure you are unlikely to be interrupted for a few minutes, get comfortable, read through the instructions in advance, and establish a relaxed, passive state of mind with the deep breathing "warm-up." Try different positions at different times (i.e., lying down, sitting, etc.); use a chair, a bed, the floor, pillows, and other props until you find the situation(s) that works just right for you. As you get skilled at this simple process of centering and quieting, you will be able to produce some of the same effects while driving, sitting in a (dull) meeting, or otherwise involved in an activity that does not require full concentration.

- Drain off excess muscle tension by rolling your head slowly in a circular fashion, first in one direction, then the other. Keep the shoulders still, and the rest of your body as relaxed as possible. Don't worry if your neck cracks and pops, so long as this is not painful and your head does not loosen or fall off your neck. Just kidding.
- Shake your hands. Let your arms hang limp for a moment, relax completely, and then shake your hands vigorously. Feel the vibration in your arms and shoulders. Do each hand separately, then together.
- Complete the deep breathing routine. This sets up a preliminary state of restful calm that facilitates a desired focus on progressive relaxation.
- Bend back your hands at the wrist. Do so slowly, until both hands are tightly drawn back as far as possible without pain. Hold this position for at least 15 seconds to the point of strain. Then release and relax, especially the wrists, hands and fingers.
- After about 30 seconds, make a tight fist with both hands. Clench your fists as hard as possible for 15 seconds. As you do this, try to relax the rest of your body. Then let go, and allow your hands to relax as fully as possible. Continue the deep breathing technique. Be sure to phase into and out of the tensing state as slowly as you can.
- Take at least three minutes to tense (hold for 15 seconds) and then, very progressively, to relax the following parts of your body in this order: your face, neck, shoulders, chest, back, stomach, legs, feet, and toes. Be attentive to

changes in your ability to concentrate upon, and alternately to tighten and loosen pressure in, each of these areas. Your level of mastery will improve as you become "better acquainted" with previously overlooked muscle groups.

· Repeat a tension-relaxation cycle of 30 seconds for any of the listed muscle groups that seemed particularly stressed or otherwise difficult to work with.

· You may choose to give further attention to an area because it seems to "hold" or call up in your mind special associations or events.

· For added effect to the letting-go phase, include a few verbalizations with the deep breathing activity. Examples are: "I release all tension in this muscle." "This area of my body is rested and peaceful." "These muscles are smooth and serene," and "all pressure in this part of my body is dissolved." Naturally, you can and should come up with phrases suited to your unique style of performing these stress-management exercises.

· Experiment with tapes that combine deep breathing and muscle relaxation,* or consider making your own. The more you put into this, the more you will get out of it.

· Work on the art of body scanning. Hospitals spend millions for high-technology, brain-scanning X-ray machines to aid in various diagnostic procedures in noninvasive ways. You can use scanning techniques, too, for free. Just let your attention pass over the parts of your body, noting the location of tight and restricted areas. Then do a relaxation number on that affected part. More areas of our bodies are subject to voluntary control than most medical authorities thought possible just a few years ago. A few doctors still are unaware of the

---

*Relaxation tapes are sold at nearly all wellness conferences, centers, and in most bookstores. The people who published this book at Whatever have a series of tapes for meditation and visualization, my favorite of which is Marcus Allen's *Stress Reduction and Creative Meditations*.

potential which their patients have for self-control and attendant natural relaxation.

· Keep a diary, ledger, or journal of how you are doing. More will be said about this come Day Fourteen; for now, just make note of occasions during the day when these rituals are most helpful, where tension was experienced, and similar observations.

Summing Up

Deep breathing and muscle relaxation are valuable used alone. However, when combined with the knowledge of stress dynamics and the wide variety of useful strategies suggested in Day Nine (plus those you come up with on your own), the results are powerful. It should now be evident that the extent of your power to manage stress is truly vast — to put it mildly. As with anything else worthwhile, it takes practice to gain mastery and to minimize the time required for good results. The payoffs are well worth the investment — which is the last point I want to make in today's lesson: namely, that while it is a very fine thing to minimize all the adverse effects of experiencing distress and tension, the greatest returns are the satisfactions in possessing these tools for personal effectiveness.

The Day is complete. Give yourself credit for another step toward wellness as an effortless and natural way of living with a dashing check after Day Ten on the *Fourteen Days* calendar.

By the way, I was really gypped yesterday. I went into a California discount massage parlor, and learned too late that it was self-service.

Cheers.

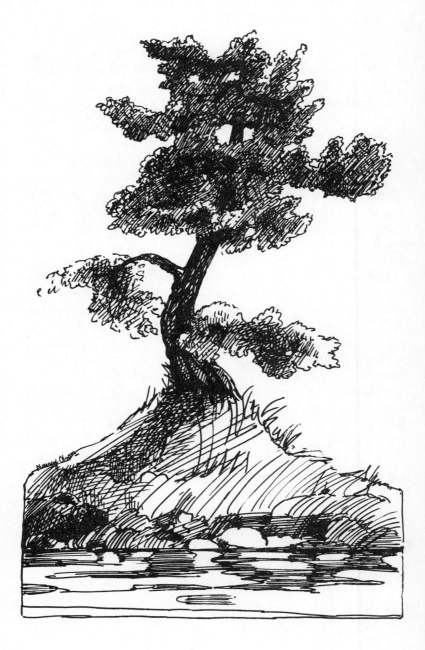

Day Eleven

Develop Visualization Skills For Relaxation, Creativity, Health Enrichment, And Personal Fulfillment

Purpose: At the end of this reading, you should want to design your own unique methods and forms for advanced stress management that provide postive outcomes. A variety of tips and visualization approaches follow which are intended to support your creativity in developing additional skills for health enhancement.

You have learned the basics about stress dynamics. You have been exposed to a variety of ways to manage stressful situations. You have a knowledge of deep breathing and muscle-relaxation techniques for dealing successfully with negative conditions while establishing calm and balance. Now it is health enhancement time — a short period of a Day's reading targeted to inner dynamics and outer payoffs or gains.

Wellness is a journey, not a destination, and visualizations make the trip more enjoyable. Though some visualization exercises may seem a little far-out at first, there is nothing really peculiar about the activity. Everybody visualizes in some fashion nearly every day. Unfortunately, few do so skillfully with wellness outcomes in mind. That is what this Day is about: learning to create and employ an untapped resource to increase the satisfactions and results of purposeful living shaped for whole-person excellence.

THE VISUALIZATION PROCESS

What is visualization? It is a way of using your conscious mind to bring about desired states, rather than simply allowing your unconscious to lead you wherever it happens to go, which is often in many directions at the same time. At one level, we all want certain things — such as love, satisfying connections with others, high-energy levels, terrific self-esteem, and so on. At another, we entertain a few programs that constantly run through our subconscious computers and get in the way — such as doubts, fear of failure, shortcomings, wrongs, and the like. Visualization can be used to quiet things, sort out the riffraff of negativity, and set you up for attractive outcomes. It is unchallenged knowledge that what goes on in the mind, such as pictures of doubt or confidence, fear or anticipation, and so on, affects not only heart rates and muscle tension, but also learning acuity, perceptions, motivations, and beliefs. Thus, the entire area is just too important to be left to chance, or to unconscious negative programming.

As usual, I'm not promoting airy-fairy practices that will make you a mystic or psychic, or lead you to take vacations in strange places with gurus having funny accents. Visualization in a wellness context will simply facilitate your efforts to sustain good lifestyle intentions while providing very enjoyable practices for stress management. Your expectations must be realistic. Fifteen minutes will not change your life. However, an openness to new techniques may very well start you on a system that allows many useful insights. Let me note a few of the advantages connected with the regular practice of visualization or use of imagery. First, it can enhance your ability to maintain a psychological and physical balance and a state of high energy in the presence of adversity or opportunity. Second, it can strengthen your capacity for self-reliance in order for you to better serve the communities you care about. Third, it can be a big help in building self-confidence and extending your learning abilities. Fourth, it can lead to dramatic increases in self-responsibility for your own health and positive outcomes in life situations. And, fifth, the process and outcome of visualization practices are usually both gratifying and enjoyable.

Remember, the *forms* employed for visualization purposes are not important. What matters are results — and your degree of satisfaction with and attendant commitment to these processes *are* basic elements of the result. If additional outcomes develop, which is highly likely, all the better.

We are just beginning to understand how ordinary people, busy getting about the myriad activities of earning a living, raising a family, and having fun, can develop these self-regulatory skills. More and more, visualization techniques are being employed by physicians, psychiatrists, and others to deal with problem areas. This entails helping people gain control over brain-wave patterns, skin temperature, heart rhythms, blood flow, and muscle action. Visualization in this context is used for pain control, disease remission, and symptom alleviation. There is, at the same time, a growing interest in what all of us can accomplish in shaping behavioral outcomes and psychological functions through the manipulation of mental processes. If visualization works to moderate suffering, then why not apply it to enhance and ennoble what has passed for "normal" experience? No reason why not, in this view. The fact that there has always been less interest in so-called health circles in health than in sickness issues need not discourage us. It is a wonderful thing that visualization works for illness treatment, pain relief, symptom control, self-regulation, altered states of consciousness, and stress disorders. All these clinical and related health-disorder applications are well and good. For Day Eleven, however, we have other objectives in mind.

Before starting, here are a few considerations on the effective use of visualization for the wellness objectives of relaxation for its own sake, added creativity, health enrichment, and personal fulfillment.

· Think of the visualization process as a special way of talking to yourself, which you do all the time anyway. An effective imagination is a more powerful tool for wellness than a storehouse of health data.

· Know that all you are really doing is developing a family of techniques to *consciously focus attention on desired positive outcomes*. At times, all of this may sound complicated, but this is what it basically comes down to.

· A vivid imagination is a birthright, effortlessly shaped in childhood but repressed and driven underground by the time most become adults. Fortunately, it can be recovered.

· Physical health is a reflection of consciousness. Lifestyle follows mindstyle. Our self-concepts affect our exercise patterns, food choices, stress-management practices, friendships, and the way we look, act, and think. Visualizations can reinforce and safeguard desired self-concepts.

· Since the body is always changing and rebuilding, mental alignment approaches can be used to guide certain desired outcomes for optimal physical health.

· Visualizations are more than *visual* pictures. The richest visualizations involve many senses. When you develop your own variations, add color, sound, light, heat, and anything else you can come up with that adds to the quality and power of your creations.

· Try a wide range of approaches. Work specifically with each of the five wellness dimensions. More important than a lot of experience is an attitude of openness to having fun doing new things.

· Always "warm up" before doing visualizations by spending a few minutes with deep breathing and muscle-relaxation exercises. A state of calm peacefulness is almost a requirement to experience the kind of imagery desired in visualization activity. This procedure will quiet the dominant, logical part of your nervous system, and make you more alert to the subtler sides of your being.

· Set aside a few minutes at certain parts of the day for trying the visualizations suggested below. The best times are probably at the beginning and end of the day; these are occasions that lend themselves to special rituals.

· Realize that your conscious mind is just one part of you, and not necessarily the dominant part. You are, in fact, so much more. Just consider for a moment the "weird" things that take place when you dream. These dreams consist of stored memories you forgot about or never knew you picked up in the first place. Usually, they were "translated" (in a fashion) without benefit of left-brain-hemisphere logical associations. Thus, your intuitions, feelings, drives, aspirations, and values are among the real playwrights of your dreams.

· To learn more about unknown, inner parts of your being, just follow four rules: (1) pay attention; (2) loosen up; (3) cultivate your intuitive, instinctive self; and (4) make visualization exercises a regular part of your life. The rest of this Day's lesson includes a few starter visualizations for just these purposes.

VISUALIZATIONS FOR WELLNESS

The first visualization is intended to give you a sense for

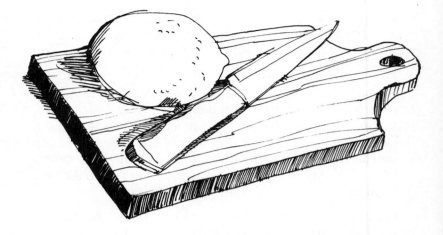

the connection between mind and body. Close your eyes (after first reading this through!). Relax your shoulders and neck. Breathe deeply. Release all tension in your muscles. Think of being in your kitchen. Notice the familiar surroundings. Feel comfortable, secure. Place three objects in front of you: a cutting board, a sharp knife, and a fresh lemon. See yourself reaching for the lemon with one hand, the knife with the other. Hold the lemon firmly against the board and slowly cut into it. In slow motion, see yourself slicing the lemon in half. Notice the pulp, the juices running off the cutting board, and the bright color of the lemon. Pay attention to the bittersweet aroma; see if you can recreate the sound of the fruit being cut. Next, select a wine glass, and squeeze the juice from half the cut lemon into the glass. Do the same with the remaining half. Now take the glass and raise it to your lips. Again, note the aroma, and whatever other details of the scene you can imagine and experience by thinking vividly about it. Begin drinking the fresh, unadulterated lemon juice, continuing to drink until the entire glass is drained. Return the glass to the table, take another deep breath, relax, and open your eyes.

What did you notice in doing this visualization? If a

friend were watching, she might observe that, at certain times, you seemed to frown, grimace, or purse your lips. Many people have such reactions. On the other hand, you may have smiled the entire time if you love lemon juice. The point of this exercise is simple: the images you create in your mind manifest feelings and behaviors expressed in that obvious part of you which others experience, and which you experience in your body, as well. Thus, by working on less evident areas of inner attunement, you move toward states that are selected and cultivated, rather than brought on (seemingly) from nowhere. Mind and body are inextricably intertwined.

Before continuing, try a brief visualization to expose lingering negatives that could be blocking your wellness paths. Imagine that you are in some courtroom setting. The jury has just returned after deliberating your case. The foreperson stands, tells the judge they are ready to unload on this sorry specimen, looks you in the eye, and says: "We find the defendant guilty of whatever it is he's accused of, and what's more we think he is dumb, lazy, mean to his animals, poor, incompetent, no fun, and selfish." Notice how you feel. Do you really believe any of these things about yourself? Which of the findings has any power over you? Thank the foreperson, the jury, and everyone else in the courtroom for helping you realize that such beliefs are ludicrous. See yourself handing the written charges to the smiling jurors, each of whom tears the copy and passes it around for more shredding. Finally, the little pieces are burned in a container, you are released from negative thoughts, and you leave the courtroom a free person, released from negative ideas about yourself.

Think about the house where you grew up. Focus your attention on one room in that house. Recall details of the scene — the color of the walls and furniture, the kinds of paintings, the rug, and other memories from long ago. Now see if you are sensing any feelings that go with these thoughts. Maintain a posture of relaxation through deep breathing and allow your imagination to carry you back to an earlier time in that house where you were little. Just notice what comes up and into conscious recall.

These are very simple, nonthreatening visualizations designed for building skill in active fantasizing. Some will work better than others. The best will come, after a bit more practice, when you start shaping your own and enjoying the activity. Remember, the rationale for visualization in Day Eleven — and in the course of a lifelong pursuit of wellness — is to increase your sense of aliveness for its own sake, not simply to deal with old upsets in a therapeutic context.

In the remaining visualizations, experiment with the use of music, particularly the selections you enjoyed most that were recommended to accompany the first ten Days. Use headphones, if available. Classical music is best, in my view, because of its melodic line and contrapuntal construction. The systematic rhythm should heighten the effects of your visualizations because it sets up aural sensations appropriate to rich feelings of well-being and harmony. The sounds from the recommended pieces by Mozart, Beethoven, Bach, and the others can travel unimpeded through the brain without resistance or reduction, and help activate a flow of stored memories. Under such conditions, your left and right hemispheres are more apt to work in harmony. Try it.

Do this next visualization lying flat on your back, legs apart, eyes closed, jaw relaxed, totally calm. Spend the usual time on the preparatory breathing and muscle-release exercises. Play Pachelbel's *Kanon,* or whatever you like.

Recall an attractive place you know well. Think of some outdoor sanctuary or refuge you greatly enjoy. Select a trail or a clearing, an overlook, or other location in a natural setting that has pleasant effects on your mood. Imagine that you are at this place. Notice the warmth of the sun on your face and chest. Feel the breeze of fresh air all around

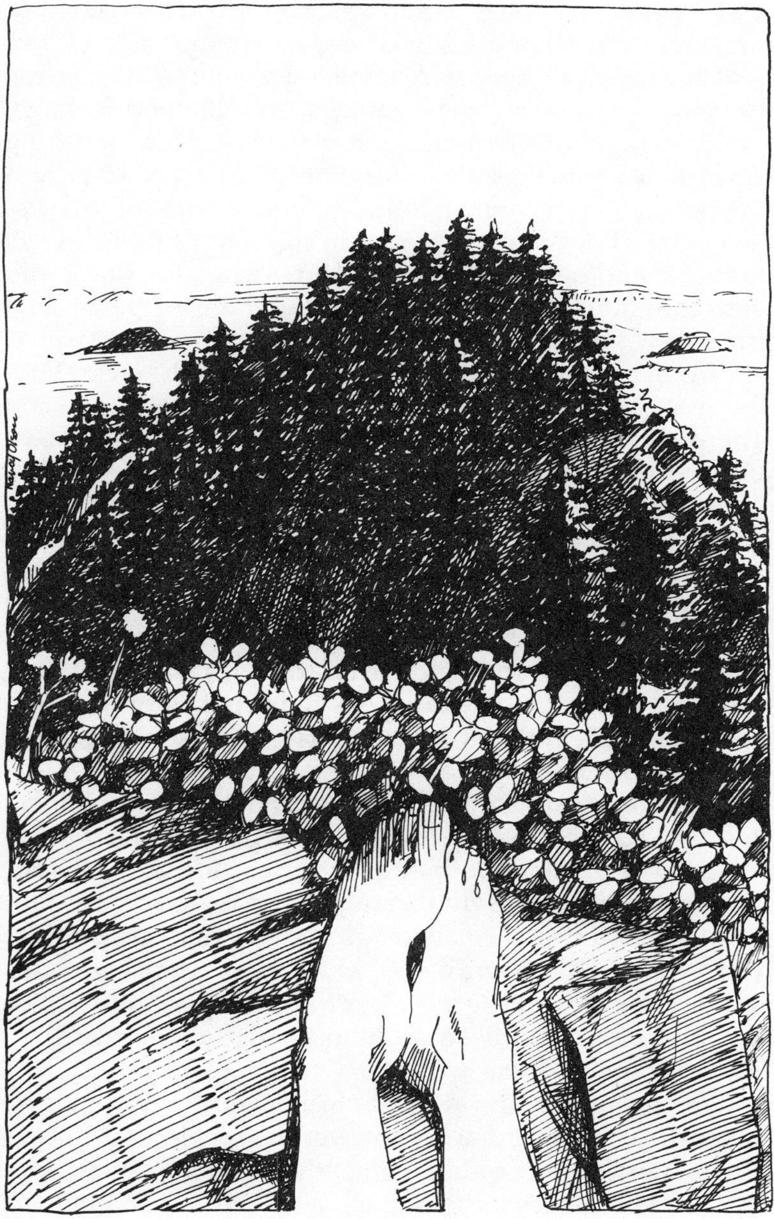

you. Smell the flowers, and the scent of berries. Listen to the ducks and other birds overhead and in the trees. Hold a leaf. Breathe very deeply. Acknowledge yourself for having the wisdom to create these images, sounds, and feelings, for knowing that there are such places, and for managing your life in a way that allows for times like this. Notice again the nourishing, energizing, and freeing quality of this visualization. Let the music soar through your brain. Just lie there for another minute or so. Allow whatever flows into your consciousness to be there. Accept these images as gifts from your inner world.

We all have a special innate wisdom, a sixth sense about things of which, on a waking level, we are largely unaware. There are visualizations to gain access to these unexplored, under-the-surface treasures. Such processes follow intuitive paths, which often require the services of an inner guide. In this visualization, introduce yourself to the guide who can show you around the inner you, unlocking treasures of insight about yourself. Be open to the idea that your guide has a great sense of humor: he, she, or it may take unexpected forms, such as an animal, a bird, a child, or a disembodied voice from above, from below, or from nowhere at all. You may simply sense — not see, feel, hear, or touch — a presence.

Prepare as usual for the visualization period. When you begin to feel that wonderful sense of peace, interconnectedness, deep experience of affection for life, and all your magnificent blessings, return to your treasured place. With gentleness, invite the source within you to come out. Let your own wellness guru feel welcome in your conscious mind. Look far out the path leading from your refuge and see the form in the distance. Notice its gradual, revealing, and welcome approach.

As the guide draws even nearer, notice your rising sense of security and acceptance of the revelation.

Acknowledge the guide; greet this master in silent, joyful tribute. Thank this benign force for the visit. Notice the good feeling, and gradually phase down the visualization. You want to avoid pressing the wellness guru, or being too pushy at the first meeting.

In a day or so, repeat this visualization. When you feel ready, give your inner guide a tour. Ask questions. Inquire if the inner guide might like to make a statement, ask a question, or get some advice. (Even inner guides need support systems for wellness.)

Your guide may be big on riddles or paradoxes. It may be very direct and to the point. Be accepting of anything. Appreciate your guide. Think of each session as complete.

Do not get trapped in a rational context that could ruin everything. Your guide need not be "real" to serve.

Call upon the guide in ways that are comfortable for you. It is not the only source of love and support, of guidance and wisdom, but it sure is a nice addition to the more traditional forms.

Another visualization you may enjoy involves super abundance. Think of something you want. If the good fairy were to tap you with her wand and let you have whatever you desire, what would it be? Maybe you can daydream of something that you usually do not allow yourself to want because it is impractical, impossible, too expensive, sinful, weird, greedy, unfair, or whatever. For five minutes, at least, you can have it all now till your soul is content. What will it be? Warm up to the process, take your time preparing, and ease into and beyond the breathing and muscle-relaxation phases.

Indulge yourself. There you are. You are fabulously endowed with that which you seek. Everyone loves you, is happy for you, marvels at your abundance, and acclaims you without reservation. Live it up; then slowly and gently come back to Earth. Note that this is a pretty good place, also.

For another wellness-oriented visualization, create the appropriate setting, serene body state, and mood of imaginative openness. This time, try a session with the magnificent you, out there at the farthest reaches of ultimate wellness. Notice the surfeit of delicious, wholesome foods which you and everyone else enjoys. Observe the fact that everyone seems fit, that people of all ages and races celebrate vigorous conditioning pursuits with grace and power. At intervals, see pauses in the activities of the day as citizens practice varied forms of stress management. Reflect on the fact that wellness is so natural and effortless in this setting of omnipresent well-being. Complete this visualization by performing an act symbolizing your awesome grandeur. Maybe Bert Parks is singing about you as you walk down a ramp in Atlantic City, crowned Ms. Galactic Cosmos or whatever befits your pulchritude. Perhaps you are being toasted at the United Nations for bringing about world peace. Perhaps you just saved the whales, charmed the Russians, liberated somebody, or helped a child. Whatever you did, it was terrific, and everybody admires you and is grateful. More important, you feel wonderful about it.

I'll close this by telling you of one of my recent visualizations. It started as a dream, but I liked it so much I decided to keep it when I awoke. It only lasted a few minutes, but was action-packed. The scene is a small town 26 miles from the Prudential Building in Boston called Hopkinton. It is Patriot's Day and noon is about to strike. It is the year 2001. Twenty thousand runners are in front of me, and we are awaiting the starter's gun to begin the 105th running of the Boston Marathon. Boom — the race is on. The superstars are off at sub-five-minute miles. I do not reach the starting line for 10 minutes. No problem. I move out effortlessly. I am enjoying the crowds. I see Johnny Kelley running his 70th Boston. I pass Bill Rodgers, Seko, and Virgin, all much older but as fast as ever. Two hours pass rapidly. I have glided through the pack as if carried along on great wings by a jetstream. I join the leaders as the turn is made down the final stretch. I glance at the two favored superstars locked in a high-speed dash to the tape. They look at me in amazement, then, each extends a hand — he on the one side, she on the other. We break the tape in unison — and tie for victory in two hours and five minutes, a world record. The other co-winners are in their early twenties; everyone wants to know how an "old" man could emerge from the pack to run so fast, so far, so powerfully.

I explain that it is all due to my wellness lifestyle. Naturally, this does wonders for book sales, and wellness becomes a way of life for everybody.

By this time, you probably have the idea. The best visualizations are homemade editions. All of these examples have been warm-ups, just samplers to get you thinking this way. Now it is time to design your own.

Visualizations for stress management are ennobling. They make life richer, improve your prospects for achieving goals, and help bring about desired conditions and states of being. One of the surest pathways to wellness is through imagination. Experiment — try tapes, detailed scenarios of various kinds, maybe even a class or workshop on the subject. But don't miss out. Visualizations are a natural high — as is the good, healthy, and complete life they help bring about.

Not so long ago, I would share my fantasies with anyone, anytime. A date might ask, quite casually, "What are you thinking about?" and I would launch into a tale about my latest visualization. Not so anymore. Today, I keep my fantasy life in the closet. Credit for this goes to a very special friend in Denver named Claire Raines. I'll never forget what she said to me one evening, with tenderness, sweetness, but unwavering honesty: "Don, dear, if people were interested in your fantasies, they would not be fantasies anymore."

Time for another check mark. On to Day Twelve — tomorrow.

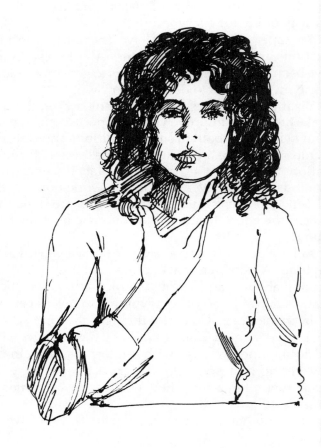

Day Twelve

Learn About And Start To Monitor Your Wellness Vital Signs

Purpose: To raise your curiosity about key measures of positive health, and to trigger an investigation into your baseline wellness status.

The focus for this Day is on tangible measures of genuine health. These measures, called wellness vital signs, will give you an accurate and revealing record of programs farther along the wellness path toward your best possibilities.

A standard physical exam is oriented to discovering signs and symptoms of illness; the existence of varying states of well-being is not part of assessing clinical history. This is a ridiculous situation. It occurs because our cultures are disease-oriented. There is great concern for stomach distress, sore throats, and headaches; there is no medical interest in stomach pleasures, throat delights, or head joys. This neglect must end. You can contribute to a new set of expectations by learning to assess how *healthy* you are. The idea is that if you know in specific ways about positive states of health (as well as negative conditions of sickness), you will gain added satisfaction over time from increases in your state of well-being.

Day 12 is set up to provide you with starter information on wellness vital signs. There are two types of positive health indicators: (1) tangible measures which are scientific, verifiable, established, dependable, and otherwise subject to objective assessment or quantification; and (2) intangible measures which have none of the above characteristics, are anecdotal, personalized, and sometimes a little far-out. Intangible measures are just as valuable as the tangible signs of positive health. You can begin now to learn about both.

Tangible Wellness Vital Signs

The first and most obvious vital sign is resting heart rate. In this country, doctors have been known to tell a patient that everything is "normal" if his or her resting heart rate is 90 beats per minute. Of course, "normal" is not a very desirable condition if the majority is unfit, as is true of North Americans generally. If everyone in your town was four feet tall, weighed 400 pounds, and was an alcoholic chain smoker, would you want to be a "normal" citizen in the community? Not likely. When the prevailing standards are far below your potentials, you can do better and reach farther than mere normalcy. This is the case with respect to resting-heart-rate standards; for example, I think you should be able to slow your resting pulse to not more than 60 beats per minute.* Heart rate is a condition of heart-muscle strength and the efficiency of blood circulation. The work being done by a resting heart beating 60 times per minute is simply more efficient and less demanding than the heart working at a higher pace. Gabe Mirkin, a noted sports-medicine physician, quotes a Northwestern University study indicating that a person with a resting heart rate

---

*The Canadian Ministry of Culture and Recreation, sponsor of the Fitness Ontario program, recommends 70 beats per minute as a standard of fitness. In a wellness context, the standard could be just a bit more challenging.

of over 80 beats a minute has five times greater risk of having a heart attack. Another study at the University of Washington Medical School showed that an 80-plus resting heart rate is one of three factors that create an 80 percent chance of death from heart disease within three years. When you become better conditioned, your heart rate will drop. While training can momentarily increase your heart rate, the improved conditioning will lower your total daily heart beats by 10,000-20,000 beats. This shows that exercise has the desired effect of changing body functions.* In simplest terms, a lower heart rate means you can do the same work with less effort for extended periods of time. With endurance-type exercise, your cardiac muscle becomes more fit. Using an analogy with the skeletal muscles, it could be said that, with exercise, your "heart-muscle physique" starts to look more like Arnold Schwarzenegger's and less like Woody Allen's.

Closely related to this wellness vital sign is heart recovery after exercise. The heart rate returns to normal in two stages after exercise at your target rate, and each stage is separated by a leveled out or stabilized plateau period of several minutes or, sometimes, much longer. According to Covert Bailey, the author of *Fit or Fat,* † neither the plateau nor the second return to normal phase is of great use for assessing your fitness level. What seems most useful for this purpose is the slope of the rate of recovery in the first minute, as charted on a graph. This is done by subtracting the pulse at one minute from the exercise pulse and dividing by 10, which gives the recovery rate. Steeper slopes get higher numbers, and are indicative of better-conditioned, healthier hearts. Using the same approach, a 30-second (first half-minute recovery) count can also be obtained (divide by five); the larger of the two slopes would be the heart recovery rate. The recovery rate values in plotting the slope are: less than two is poor fitness; two to three is fair; three to

---

*Per-Olaf Astrand, *Health and Fitness* (Stockholm, Sweden: Skandia Insurance Company, Universaltryck: 1972), pp. 14-15.

†Covert Bailey, *Fit or Fat* (Boston: Houghton-Mifflin Co., 1978).

four is good; four to six is excellent; and more than six is super. If all this is too complicated, relax. Here's a simpler method. Just count your pulse for 10 seconds immediately after stopping exercise. Multiply by six. Wait one minute. Repeat the 10 count. Your pulse should have come down at least 25 beats per minute. If not, you are in poor shape. Notice the difference in this recovery rate as you become better conditioned.

A third wellness vital sign is a one-second forced expiratory volume (FEVI) test. This provides a measure (in liters of air) of respiratory (lung) function. This respiratory function test, along with a related vital capacity assessment, is available in most fitness centers, YMCAs, hospitals, and health centers. You breathe into a machine, which registers the amount of air you are able to exhale in a unit of time. You are assigned a score, calculated as a percentage of the capacity which can be predicted for a person of your age and body size. For persons interested in knowing how far out to the right they are on the positive side of the Worseness/Wellness Continuum, this indicator is of special value. In combination with oxygen uptake, it is indicative of how fully you take in and utilize oxygen, how well that oxygen is transferred to the blood, and how effectively carbon-dioxide wastes are expelled from the lungs. Lung-function and oxygen-uptake tests will also give former smokers and others at risk a reading concerning the degree to which his/her airways are open for the passage of gas, the extent of constrictions (e.g., asthma), lost elasticity (e.g., emphysema), and mucus (e.g., as in chronic bronchitis or "smokers cough"). The tests are inexpensive, quick, painless, and interesting (you can see a graph of your performance as you exhale into the spirometer). Pulmonary function tests provide accurate estimates of your respiratory efficiency. If you are fit, you should be able to average at least five liters of air in a single breath (FEVI), an indicator that you can sustain a higher percentage of your maximum breathing capacity for longer time periods. In other words, your lungs are able to support the availability of large amounts of oxygen needed for strenuous exercise.

The standards of predictive values are related to your height, sex, and age. From a wellness perspective, you probably will not be satisfied with less than 80 percent of predicted value in order to participate in your chosen exercise routines free of respiratory impairment.

A forced exhalation volume test is a useful measure of the elasticity of your lungs and breathing tubes. Unlike other wellness vital signs, your performance level in the lung test probably will not show appreciable differences in six months to a year, even if you do pursue a vigorous wellness lifestyle. For better or worse, it took many years to condition your respiratory system to be where it is today; it may be many years from the start of a conditioning program before you are able to develop your FEVI capacity to the point you desire. Still, it is good to know where you stand on this right side of the continuum, positive health indicator. In short, this vital sign is about how well you breathe. The good news is that your capacity to utilize oxygen can actually be increased through trainings by as much as 20 percent.

Most people know, more or less, what they weigh; very few know how much of their body is fat versus how much is lean mass (muscle, bone, fluid, skin, and organ weight). For the majority interested only in understanding if they are sick or likely to become so, percent of body fat is of little interest. This situation is not surprising or unreasonable. However, persons like yourself who are more interested in moving to the right of the Worseness/Wellness Continuum toward optimal health will benefit from knowing how and why to monitor this fourth wellness vital sign.

Your body has two basic kinds of tissue, adipose (fat) and lean body (muscle and bone). An excess of the former increases the energy requirements which you need for everyday tasks, and all your bodily systems must operate at higher levels. The result is that you stress your body more than is necessary, day after day. An appropriate ratio of fat to lean muscle mass enables you to function more efficiently, and is associated with added protection against heart disease, high blood pressure, diabetes, and lower back problems.

The desired range for adult males and females is not universally agreed upon, but the following percentages are representative of what most exercise physiologists utilize for excellent to poor ratings:

	Males	*Females*
Excellent	15% or less	18% or less
Good	18% to 21%	20% to 23%
Average (normal!)	20% to 24%	24% to 27%
Poor	25% or higher	28% or higher

Fat, like stress, is inevitable and desirable. Fat is one means by which your body stores energy, protects the vital organs, and gains insulation against heat loss. As with stress, however, too much of a good thing, without awareness of the build-up and without action to control and modify the intake, is hazardous both to your natural desire for illness avoidance and your prospects via wellness for superhealth. An excess of fat means obesity and a dozen or more unpleasant, dysfunctional conditions that do you no good and a lot of harm.

Ever hear someone say, "I lost twenty pounds!"? The logical response from someone who knows about this wellness vital sign, would not be "Congratulations," but something like "Twenty pounds of what?" If you diet without exercise, you lose lean muscle tissue as well as excess or storage fat. Diet alone is not effective in reducing intramusculature fat; at best it temporarily removes some subcutaneous (below the skin) fat along with muscle tissue (which you do not want to lose). There ought to be a law or at least a consumer advisory against diet books that contain not a word about exercise. Anyone who knows about this wellness vital sign will never fall prey to the "pound foolish" trap. It is not what you weigh that really matters — it's how much fat you have that counts. To the trash bin with the bathroom scale — it does more harm than good by putting an exclusive focus on body weight.

So, how much fat *should* you have if you are as physically fit as you would like to be or, more important, as you expect yourself to be as you approach optimal conditioning? You should definitely expect that, eventually, you will move into the "excellent" category as noted above. That is, not more than 15 percent of your body should consist of fat, if you are male, 18 percent if female. Naturally, you will not meet this test without a regular fitness program of some kind. Average readings at executive health retreats are about 24 percent for males, 29 percent for females. These are probably better than general public averages, since conferees at these workshops go to considerable time and expense to attend the programs, and thus are probably a little better motivated than most. Of course, *average* is not even a respectable standard, since most people seldom move to the right side of the neutral point on the Worseness/Wellness Continuum.

A further comment on our nonexistent but statistically useful *average* representative Joe or Jane seems warranted. Being sedentary, he or she will put *on* about a pound of fat per year after age 25, so that at age 55, Mr. or Ms. Average is going to be 30 pounds (of fat) heavier. However, about a half-pound of muscle and bone will also be *lost* each year due to inactivity, and will be replaced by fat. So, figure on another 15 pounds of fat taking the place of lean muscle tissue. Thus, while the actual scale weight of our *normal* or average model citizen will be 30 pounds greater on the bathroom scale, the net gain of *fat* is actually 45 pounds. The individual, unfortunately, will only know about the 30 pounds of weight gain — unless he or she knows about and monitors this wellness vital sign. If not, he/she remains blissfully unaware that body composition has shifted dramatically, and dangerously. The person now weighs (at least) 30 pounds more than is desirable and, more significantly, has lost 15 pounds of critical lean muscle tissue.

You have a significant advantage in knowing about this vital sign, because the opposite effect occurs with exercise in combination with caloric reduction; the major portion of weight loss is in fat tissue rather than lean muscle mass. Exercise protects the lean tissue as you become a more efficient burner of fat, and more muscle tissue helps you in this regard. Lower body fat means better muscle tone, improved muscle chemistry and higher metabolic rates, meaning that you burn more calories in whatever you do (including relaxing and sleeping). The benefit of maintaining a low percent of body fat means you are more effective at delivering oxygen and burning fat.

This wellness vital sign is best measured in a device called a hydrostatic tank, or immersion tank. You sit in a hot tub-like device, exhale to the maximum extent, and allow your entire body to go underwater. Your weight is taken and, using conversion tables for weight, height, sex and age, a calculation of body composition is made. The technique is based on Archimedes' observation that the volume of an object is determined by its loss of weight in water. In other words, fat floats, muscle sinks or weighs more. As Bailey has observed, for purposes of body composition, dense is beautiful. The more you weigh underwater, the less fat and more muscle mass you have. Another less accurate but more widely available and quite useful indicator of body composition is the hand calipers, which allows a tester to calculate fat- and muscle-tissue ratios by a series of skin-fold measurements. Another version of the skin-fold caliper, calibrated in millimeters rather than percentages, and organized in categories (e.g., "lean, ideal, average, and obese"), is the fat-control device.* Any

---

*The fat caliper and instruction booklet is available from Fat Control, Inc., P.O. Box 10117, Towson, MD 21204. The price is $8.95 prepaid.

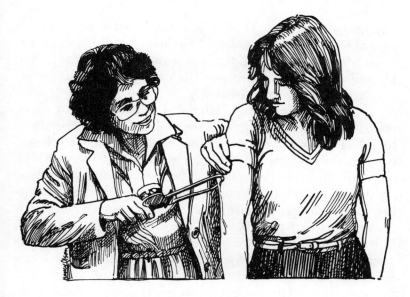

method is desirable, in my view. Just be sure to have it done.

There are two major payoffs in knowing this wellness vital sign: (1) it gives you a superb indicator of genuine progress if you know what your body composition is *before* you begin a serious exercise regimen; and (2) it is a highly reliable indicator of optimal physical well-being.

While not a substitute for a body-*fat* test, you can get an idea of where you are in relation to an ideal body *weight* by using the following formula. For males, multiply your height in inches by 4.0 and subtract 128; for females, multiply your height in inches by 3.5 and subtract 108. (The formula is for adults with medium body frames. If your bone structure is unusually large or small, you will have to invent your own formula!)

Target heart rate (THR) is the next wellness vital sign I would like you to know about. As you recall from the discussion of the intensity measure of adequacy in Day 7 devoted to physical fitness, THR is a measure of the level of effort required to obtain the best returns from exercise. If you know what your THR is, you almost surely are knowledgeable regarding how best to achieve cardiovascular fitness. More important, if you know about THR, you probably are already getting better than adequate regular exercise, and benefiting accordingly.

You can compute your THR using a standard forumla, or you can have your exact rate figured on an exercise-stress test. The stress test involves time, expense, and hard work, but it is the best measure available. To calculate your THR using the formula, proceed as follows: take 220 (theoretical maximum heart rate) minus your age (some favor substituting your resting heart rate instead of your age). This is your maximum heart rate. Next, take 70 percent of this value. This is your one-minute heart rate for aerobic-exercise purposes. Divide this last figure by 6, or the amount of time required in a 10-second count to have a pulse in the 70 percent range. The 10-second figure is your exercise rate. For best results, exercise as you wish but monitor your 10-second count until (in a short time) you know what your body feels like when it is in the target zone.

Not everyone should start out at this rate, nor should everyone remain at this level indefinitely. For those out of condition or concerned about a possible heart irregularity or similar problem. some pre-exercise testing followed by exercise at 60-65 percent of maximum may be preferable. For persons in average condition, a range from 65-75 may be the best approach. For those in excellent shape, target zones in the 75-85 percent range will provide better results.

However, if this is too mathematical for you, consider the simple formula for pulse-rate goals given in Day 7.

Again, you would not want to interrupt your aerobic exercise to take a 60-second count, so calculate your 10-second count or exercise rate. A simpler, not quite as accurate but valid method is to count for six seconds (starting with zero) and add a zero to your count at the six-second mark. As in other wellness dimensions, the pursuit of optimum health puts you on closer terms with your own body — you become expert at reading its subtle clues regarding ups and downs, peaks and occasional valleys, and acting accordingly.

The other wellness vital signs to know are your range of motion (or flexibility quotient) and your strength level. Both are standards of adequacy discussed in Day 7. Both apply as wellness vital signs. By maintaining a high level of flexibility and muscle strength, you can perform at higher levels without unduly stressing your body. You cannot only avoid a myriad of problems associated with vigorous exercise (stiff muscles, joint disorders, lower-back pain, torn muscle fibers, damaged tendons and connective tissue), but actually derive satisfaction from these exercises. There are no universal tests or standards for assessing the precise extent of positive health in these areas, but you can get an idea by performing a few simple postures and routines. In each case, move gently and without pain or facial grimace. (The test of your present degree of flexibility and strength is not as important as your commitment to improve.) Three popular stretches are: (1) reach for your toes from a standing position without bending your legs; (2) perform five sit-ups with your hands locked behind your neck, knees bent, and both feet flat on the floor (unassisted); and (3) with legs flat on the floor in a sitting position, stretch forward and grasp your toes with both hands. Useful strength tests include push-ups, pull-ups, and hand-grip measures. How well you can perform these basic tests of flexibility and strength is another sign of how far out to the right of the scale you are on the Worseness/Wellness Continuum. In addition to all the problems you can avoid, you will find daily stretching to be a quieting activity and an important adjunct to deep-breathing and muscle-relaxation exercises.

Awareness and monitoring of these tangible wellness vital signs are prerequisites to major progress. It can be very satisfying to notice how, over time, each measure gets better as you advance toward your own potentials.

In a way, these signs are to wellness what wellness is to your overall well-being — a trump card that gives you a special edge on the rest of the world, to be used for your own purposes as well as in service to others.

My own signs have been getting better in the past two years since I started keeping track of them while pursuing a sub-two-hour and 40-minute marathon. For illustration purposes, I'm willing to share my vital signs, but do not think that you must have similar results. Depending upon your age, sex, inherent capabilities, motivations, and various lifestyle considerations, higher or lower ratings will be more appropriate for you. You are, after all, extraordinary, and your interests are best served by setting your own standards. So, with that caveat, here are my own vital sign indicators. The ratings are based on tests at Covert Bailey's mobile clinic, the Sun Valley Health Institute, the Boeing Corporation, a Seventh Day Adventist evaluation booth in Los Angeles during a public-health conference, and the North Cascade Wellness Institute. (If you do not like the results at one place, try another.)

Heart rate (beats per minute)	40
Heart recovery rate — ½ minute	9.4
1 minute	6.2
One-second forced expiratory volume (FEV — actual)	5.68
FEVI (predicted — based on age/sex/height)	4.27
Percent of predicted	133%
Forced vital capacity (FVC — actual)	6.85
FVC (predicted — based on age/sex/height)	5.62
Percent of predicted	122%
Percent of body fat	9.5%
Target heart rate	162
Weight	166
VO2/KG	64.0

You can get as much value in learning about your weaknesses in wellness areas as your strengths. As you fully realize, there *are* other measures that can be and are used to assess illness and health levels (e.g., high- and low-density lipoproteins, blood pressure, cholesterol, triglycerides, etc.). In the future, far more sophisticated tangible vital signs will help us monitor our physical well-being from the wellness part of the continuum.

There may, for example, soon be a battery of assessments that measure the "fitness level" of organ functions, cellular strength, and molecular configuration. Someday, advanced wellness vital signs will serve as "biomarkers" of aging, replacing today's arbitrary indicator of simple chronological age.* In the meantime, start keeping track of today's version of tangible wellness vital signs. They provide positive and dramatic watershed indicators of your advances toward the physical excellence that is within your reach and is part of your birthright.

Intangible Wellness Vital Signs

All the signs just described are objective, measurable indicators. Unlike much of what transpires in discussing and experiencing wellness, these signs are "scientific," not anecdotal, "soft," or dependent upon personal assessments and interpretations. But, therein lies a problem. It means that a lot of signs and indicators of positive health have been omitted because they are not measurable.

Good news. You can have it both ways. You can track the objective measures *and* pay attention to personal indicators that might be even more significant as to how healthy and truly well you are at any given time.

Here are a few such indicators:
· Energy levels at certain times of day — such as upon awakening.

---

*For a related account on vital signs and aging, see *Runner's World*, May 1981, pp. 37-40.

- Skin tone, clarity of eyes, sense of taste, etc.
- Appetites (including sexual).
- Serum fun level — are you having a good time, feeling on purpose throughout most of the day, etc.
- Dream quality and soundness of sleep.

These characteristics are not easily measured. Your assessment of them is necessarily subjective, but they are no less useful to you for indicating how you are doing in moving toward the wellness end of the continuum. What other indicators do you think might be useful? Add your own — it cannot do any harm and will surely serve to raise your conscious awareness of health as more than not being sick.

Summary

Now you know what doctors should look for in medical checkups. Wouldn't it be a neat idea if schools, businesses, hospitals, and other institutions and private clubs encouraged their members to fully appreciate why such positive indicators are important to track over time. They could even provide the facilities and programs that make such tracking easy, inexpensive, and interesting. Well, you do not have to wait for the millenium or hoped-for era of prosperity, justice, and enlightenment to learn of the importance of wellness vital signs. You just learned all about them in Day 12.

For now, just be conscious of these superb indicators of positive health. Just to know why they are important is an improvement; contrast where you are now with the idea of simply thinking of health as the absence of illness or disease.

Do not be discouraged if you think you are fat. You are not! At the moment, you may be underheight for your weight, that's all.

I enjoy giving lectures on wellness vital signs and other

aspects of the wellness lifestyle. Last month, I gave the keynote address to the Philadelphia Society of Manic Depressives. I was terrific. One minute, I had them laughing in the aisles; the next, I had them in tears.

Check Day 12 — congratulations on your progress and commitment.

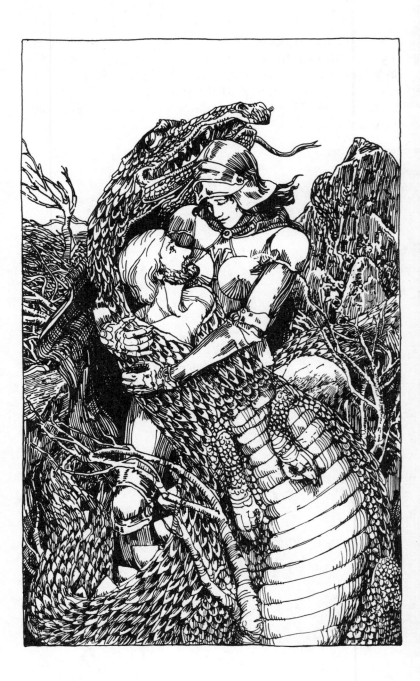

Day Thirteen

Entertain The Notion Of Becoming A Hero

Purpose: The purpose of this Day is to have you seriously entertain the idea of planning for and eventually undertaking a heroic act. This idea is admittedly far-out. It may not be for you. It is strictly optional. During this Day, I define what I mean by heroic act, what "heroism" is and what it is not, and the dangers, safeguards, requirements, implications, forms, and the payoffs associated with such endeavors. In addition, I throw in a few vignettes from my interviews with heroes, and provide you with a little test to help you decide if a heroic act is likely to appeal to you and work for you. In short, there are two purposes for Day 13: (1) to entertain you with what I hope you decide is an interesting idea (even though you may conclude that such "extremism" is impractical or not appropriate or desirable for you); and (2) to demonstrate how initiatives in one area of wellness living complement and reinforce both your commitment to and satisfactions from wellness in other areas. Enjoy — this is a special Day.

HEROISM DEFINED

A recent participant in what some consider the ultimate marathon — the Western States 100 Mile Run, held each year near Lake Tahoe in California's Sierra Nevada mountains — was asked for a comment upon completing the event in just under the twenty-four-hour limit. The exhausted runner, reflecting upon a hot day and a cold night of struggles over rugged trails, through streams and heavy brush, over snow and rocks, exclaimed with a mixture of triumph and dismay, "I wouldn't trade this experience for a million dollars. And I wouldn't do it again for two million."

You might be thinking that I have gone off the deep end — that in less than two weeks I am going to try to persuade you to run an ultramarathon, swim the English channel, bike across Canada, or do some other damn fool activity. Not so. Well, at least not exactly.

By heroic act, I mean any physical activity that you complete after a lengthy period of strenuous preparation. It is heroic in the sense of endurance and commitment required to prepare for and eventually complete the climactic act, not in the sense of derring-do or macho risktaking.

The thesis to consider today is that such an endeavor might strengthen your inner resources, offer a high degree of personal satisfaction, and continually reinforce your wellness perspective on life. Through a process of interviews, a literature search, and mail surveys, I have come to suspect that heroic acts often provide the mental strength needed to engage, sustain, and escalate a wellness lifestyle. In the course of such pursuits, there is a good chance that you could experience even more pleasure and meaning, love and worth, and zest for life than you already enjoy.

Please realize that what I am calling a heroic act can take many forms. In every case, however, it is associated with going the distance, overcoming obstacles of mind and heart, and achieving an aura of personal legend and mystery once reserved for statesmen, movie stars, and super-jocks. Heroic acts are not about running marathons (though that is one form available) or finding a magic bullet (panacea) for wellness. As emphasized, such acts are not necessarily for everyone. It is perfectly possible to pursue wellness without such endeavors. The idea of a heroic act is just that — an idea. It is not a detailed proposal or blueprint; it has not been scientifically proven through double blind cross-over trials; it is not a shortcut to *Nirvana*. Most important, it is no substitute for a balanced and integrated life guided by vision and purpose.

A heroic act *is* about escalating a wellness lifestyle. By having you consider, for this Day, the possibility of *someday* pursuing an aerobic or endurance type of fitness activity for an extended period, you will be in a position later on (say, for instance, tomorrow) to determine whether such an effort will contribute toward your goals for wellness living.

Examples of heroic act forms that have played important roles in the wellness lifestyles of persons I have studied include long distance swims, bike touring, epic hikes, cross-country ski racing, marathon and other distance runs, and a few martial arts.

Approached properly, a heroic act can motivate people to perceive wellness as the kind of game sketched in Day One in which they always win, find meaning, and experience recurring satisfaction. Pursued properly, it can help people set things up so they experience their lives as being whole, complete, and sufficient. In short, such an act helps people motivate themselves to change their viewpoint about consciously participating in shaping their own health. For these reasons, this notion may be of special interest to you.

THE PAYOFFS OF HEROISM

There appear to be five major payoffs attendant upon heroic acts. The first is that it creates direct incentives for the individual to make advances in the other four wellness dimensions. Regarding *personal responsibility*, for example, it soon becomes evident in carrying out the "act" that it is up to you. There is no future risk-sharing or guaranteed fallback positions — you rise or crash on your merits and particularly on the adequacy of your preparations. (Contrast this with the "health" insurance scam, where there is no incentive for personal accountability since any kind of sickness, however brought about, is equally subsidized, and good health is ignored and never rewarded.)

Concerning *nutritional awareness*, participants in heroic acts discover payoffs beyond disease avoidance. Anyone seeking maximum performance from her or his body learns soon enough that a natural food pattern high in complex carbohydrates and low in fat gives an advantage over a "standard" diet. Similarly, the value of *stress awareness and management* is appreciated in the context of competition, even if that "competition" is with herself or himself. Stress must be channeled and not allowed to create energy drains. Deep breathing, muscle relaxation, and visualization skills are invaluable in this context. Also, when a person is devoting an hour or more daily in preparation for some event, that exercise in itself serves as a release for a lot of everyday stress.

Finally, there are positive repercussions of heroic acts for the wellness dimension of *environmental sensitivity*. Whatever the forms involved (e.g., running, biking, swimming, etc.), there are always support groups available, and their importance in training is soon apparent.

Thus, the first specific advantage of a heroic act as a component of a wellness repertoire is that it beneficially affects all the other dimensions of whole-person living. It has a lever, or what Buckminster Fuller has termed a "trim tab" effect, on a wellness lifestyle. (A trim tab is a small device, about finger size, that turns the immense rudders which change the course of great ships and planes.) A heroic act, in other words, produces leverage for the practitioner of wellness that facilitates results far greater than one could normally expect given the modest energy expended. And, this is just the first benefit of a heroic act.

A second payoff associated with heroic acts as part of a wellness lifestyle is that they lead to a breakdown in your sense of limits. You find that old horizons become new foregrounds — you genuinely surprise yourself at how much you can do. Heroic acts, therefore, undermine mediocrity.

A third benefit is that it distracts from, discourages, and nearly eliminates the possibility of continuing any truly ridiculous high-risk habits. It would be hard if not impossible to maintain a negative addiction to cigarettes, alcohol, or drug abuse in the midst of a daily quest for physical excellence.

A fourth advantage is that a heroic act commitment provides a buffer against disappointments. Small and even not so small upsets, setbacks, and reverses are moderated when the quest is valued, when current gains must be protected, and when new advances are required. Specifically, when a certain advanced level has been reached and an upset occurs (e.g., you turn on the TV and all the stations are showing emergency evacuation routes out of the city), you are not likely to stew in a funk for days and allow the deterioration that would go with inactivity or depression. It may not be fun, at first, but you will keep moving in consideration of the larger returns in the distance. (This is in contrast to the motivation of the old sage of baseball, Satchell Paige, who counseled forward movement without looking back because, in his words, "somethin' may be gainin' on you.")

The fifth and final payoff I want to credit to a heroic act is that it provides, after a time, a regular and predictable occurrence of emotional highs. These highs, in turn, become addictive to those who experience them. This, of course, sustains and reinforces the endeavor, which accounts for much of the tenacity so often attributed to those who dedicate themselves to an activity and refuse to be deterred from their daily rituals by inconveniences and occasional hardships.

REQUIREMENTS

It seems to me that seven factors can be identified as requirements for the addictive effects of heroic acts to set in and for the noted payoffs to occur. These requirements are as follows:

1. The motivation must be of an internal nature. Competition is fine, even helpful to many, but it seems critical that the locus of assessment regarding performance as well as the level of satisfaction come from within.
2. The heroic act must require the individual to extend herself or himself — it must not be easy, or progress and ultimate achievement might be taken for granted.
3. The activity should provide aerobic or endurance-type cardiovascular training benefits.
4. The minimal time period of preparation for the effects to occur seems to be not less than six months, and is more likely closer to one year.
5. A clear end-phase or climactic event should be in the mind of the practitioner, in order that milestones or bench marks can be reached along the way toward goal achievement. These provide a measure of progress and a source of encouragement.
6. The desire to maximize gains must be more pervasive than an interest in minimizing losses.
7. The heroic act is partly an indicator of the individual's style and orientation to the full and exciting life, with acceptance of the risks connected with tracking in the fast lane.

SUPERHEROES

Heroic acts meeting these requirements take many forms, as I have noted. Do not think that these behaviors are open only to the minigods of fitness among us, such as Dianne Nyad (recently swam continuously for 41 hours and 49 minutes); Don Ritchie (ultramarathoner who holds the 100-mile-run record of 11 hours and 51 minutes — a seven-minute-per-mile pace!); and John Kelley (the two-time winner of the Boston Marathon who last year ran a 3-hour marathon at age 70!). You don't have to be ultra-extraordinary to become plain old extraordinary! There are people in all walks of life performing heroic acts, and finding that such endeavors are superb pathways to a wellness lifestyle. Remember, I am not urging you to adopt some such activity, but to ponder the possibilities.

TESTIMONIALS

The comments of some "heroes" whom I have interviewed or read about may be of interest in sensing how exciting and even momentous such pursuits can be for "ordinary" people like you and me. An ultramarathoner named Sixto Linares was recently quoted in a running magazine explaining why he runs 50-mile races: "If I never try anything, I never learn anything. If I never take a risk, I stay right where I am. If I hold myself back, I trade appearances for the opportunity to find out how far I can go."

Another said: "When you accomplish something like this, you won't give up on other things in your life, either. You get to feeling that there are not many things you can't do. You don't put limitations on yourself."

One investigator (of the ultra-event phenomenon), in response to a suggestion that perhaps some people who accomplish heroic acts are masochistic, states that just the opposite is true. The drive for such endeavors comes instead from "a love of life and a desire to live to the fullest extent."[*]

It is as if such people were out to defy the inevitable

---

[*]Candice Hogan, "Carousel of the Mind," *The Runner Magazine*, May 1980, p. 52.

passage of time by participating intensively in a "long series of moments."

PREPARATION

How should you prepare for a heroic act, assuming just for the fun of it that you would ever want to do such a thing? What can be learned from those who seem to have gained the most from heroic enterprises? Quite a lot, it turns out. Based on the interviews, five lessons stand out. First, accept the idea of possible failure as a necessary risk, for the presence of uncertainty may actually be an essential part of ultimate mastery. Second, think of obstacles and momentary letdowns as harbingers of future breakthroughs. Many report that their best performances followed periods of disappointment or stagnation. Third, use imagery and visualization techniques to make the goal enjoyable and achievable. By seeing yourself reveling in the prosperity of goal attainment, you increase your sense of competence and confidence. Fourth, conceive of the heroic act in manageable parts. Mentally divided into segments, epic feats seem more manageable and less intimidating. Finally, know that an activity that gives you private satisfaction is more rewarding over time than any effort oriented to public credit. In summary, the heroic act works best at the level of personal expression and satisfaction, not outer acclaim or glory.

DANGERS

There are hazards connected with heroic acts. You may get rigid about your training and injure yourself. This often happens to people who get addicted to running, and who fail to recognize messages from their bodies to go slow or lay off for a while. You could lose interest in other aspects of your life that you do not consider very heroic by comparison, such as your job, profession, family, relationships, or avocations. Your grip on reality could be loosened. Some have noted a tendency to get carried away with the "intoxication power" of certain activities to the point of thinking themselves indestructible supermen. In a *Sports Illustrated* story about the hazards of excessive jogging, the following account of "illusory omnipotence" was given:

> One day last spring I was having an exceptionally good run. I was running about 10 miles a day at the time and on this particular day I had decided to extend my workout. I was around the 14-mile point, and I was preparing to cross a one-lane bridge when, all of a sudden, a large cement mixer turned the corner and began to cross the bridge. I never thought for a second about stopping and letting the truck pass. I simply continued and said to myself, "Come on, you son of a bitch, I'll split you right down the middle, there'll be concrete all over the road!" The driver slammed on the brakes and swerved to the side of the road as I sailed by. That was really *scary* afterward, but at the time it felt really *good!**

If this were not enough, there is yet another possible hazard: you may find yourself thinking of persons not engaged in such eminent pursuits of a conditioning nature as "moral slugs" — or worse. This would be unfortunate for reasons beyond the essential inaccuracy of such an outlook. If you think you are living in the pits with the turkeys, it is hard to imagine yourself soaring the heavens like an eagle.

SAFEGUARDS

Fortunately, there are surefire safeguards against these hazards. For starters, an obvious protection is forewarning, which you now enjoy. Only a small percentage of perfor-

---

*William Oscar Johnson, "Marching to Euphoria," *Sports Illustrated,* July 14, 1980, pp. 81-82.

mers of great deeds of fitness ever lose touch with the rest of life, anyway. To be extra cautious, however, keep a few guides in mind if you do entertain the notion of a heroic act.

The first is to loosen up — do not worry about missed workouts. Have alternate activities available for those times when injury or time constraints (travel, business opportunities, friendship requirements) get in the way. If you are positively addicted to your heroic act, these substitutes can be Methadone-like alternatives. The second guide is not to take the temperature every day, a remark Henry Kissinger offered on diplomacy. There will be days when you perform poorly. Expect downs as well as ups, and you will not be surprised. Third, be charitable toward sedentary folks with unpleasant habits. Do not think poorly of others, both as a courtesy to them (you would be in the same situation if exposed to like influences and circumstances), and as a protection for your own serenity. Fourth, relish and work on developing even more the value of flexibility. Have creative and multiple options beyond the heroic act as life purposes.

I doubt, given your interest in a balanced lifestyle, that you would need to remind yourself of these precautions, but now that you know, you need them even less!

WHY DO HEROIC ACTS SERVE?

I can only speculate on the reasons why heroic acts have the effect of strengthening one's inner resources, and why such acts performed regularly over a period of time lead to the benefits described. Perhaps there is some basis in human physiology that accounts for the addiction and mental highs. Maybe long hours of repetitious training develop reserves of imagination and unusual perseverance, extending one's capacity for sustaining long-range-goal quests. Perhaps such a discipline makes immediate-need gratifications less tempting. Whatever is going on, it is clear that fulfillment, though postponed, is indeed glorious when it arrives at the time a heroic act is completed. Some say the sensation is not even available through other means. Though expensive in a time sense, the price paid is usually perceived as a bargain.

The likeliest explanation is in terms of intrabody chemistry. It seems our brains release a substance called endorphins during vigorous and sustained exercise. This substance, a part of the neurotransmitter system of our bodies, is akin to morphine in that it deadens pain and introduces a sense of euphoria.

A HEROIC ACT IN YOUR FUTURE?

This gives you a broad picture of the what, why, and how of heroic acts. Maybe it is for you, maybe not. Here are a few questions you can ask yourself to elicit some thoughts and feelings on the matter. Just play with the idea for now.

- Do you enjoy some kind of physical activity? I mean, *really* enjoy it?
- Do you feel your level of participation in some physical activity of your choice is less than you would like it to be? What if you had more time to devote to developing your talents or indulging your special interests?
- If you were to pursue such a quest for at least a year, can you think of what your choice of activity might be?
- Have you noticed that you admire people who have accomplished something that, as discussed here, amounts to a heroic act?
- Do you think you have the physical capability to undertake and see through all the challenges involved in pursuing an extraordinary feat of endurance and perseverance?
- Do you believe that just about anyone has the innate capability to perform a vigorous program over a long period of time if he or she chooses to do so?

- Can a heroic act be undertaken without sacrificing a well-rounded, integrated wellness lifestyle?
- Have you ever done anything like the kind of act described?
- Do you think you have the capacity to do so, if you wanted to?
- Do you enjoy time alone?
- Do you ever wonder what your limits might be in any activity or sport?
- Have you ever thought, when reading about someone's special achievement that, there but for _____, that might have been me?
- Are you more oriented to and motivated by personal satisfactions than by a need or desire to please others?
- Are there any undesirable habits that you might eradicate or diminish if you had a special goal that required your best efforts, day after day, for an extended period?
- Do you know people who have pursued or are now engaged in what has herein been described as a heroic act?
- The last question is this: If you came to a narrow bridge and found yourself face to face with an oncoming cement mixer, would you move aside?

If you answered yes to the great majority of these questions, that is an indicator in my view that you would do quite nicely by adding a heroic act to your wellness repertoire. Of course, once having had the experience, you may conclude that you would not repeat the endeavor for two million dollars, either. But, such good and treasured memories!

In my experience as a marathon runner, I have sensed that a heroic act offers a great buffer against, and a new perspective on, life crises, as well as helpful perspective during advances. The best moments in our lives occasionally follow the toughest problems, the biggest sacrifices, and the worst setbacks.

The pursuit of a heroic act can never guarantee the gains described. It can only provide the opportunity for personal challenge and renewal, a chance to test yourself, and maybe a time to find new levels of power, grace, and achievement. I remember the comment of one hero: "... this achievement was my theatre of distinction, a stage with all the classic elements of drama. I loved it — it gave me nobility."

George Bernard Shaw described nobility as "purpose recognized by ourselves as mighty." The best thing about the heroic act idea may be that it removes nobility from the exclusive domain of the fitness minigods like the Nyads, Ritchies, and Kelleys, and puts it within the reach of everyone. There is the possibility that it is better to attempt too much than it is to venture too little. After all, as Browning would observe if he were around today: "A man or woman's reach should exceed his/her immediate grasp, else what's a heaven for?"

IT REALLY WORKS!

You are missing out if you do not know someone who has achieved her or his goal during the quest of some heroic act. My files are rich with inspirational case histories; the following letter excerpt will give you a sense for what it is like when you *really* defy the idea of moderation.

I am a 44-year-old female, married for 22 years, and have spent 20 of those years as a housewife and mother to four children, now ages 21, 19, 17, and 14. I have never been much of an athlete, since girls were not encouraged in sports when I was young. However, I have always been an active rather than passive person, and have a lot of energy (which was in full demand with four small children).

At the age of 39, I was approached by a neighbor who wanted to start jogging, and so we began together — this was 5½ years ago. We worked up to two miles a day, and continued at that distance for two years.

When a group of running friends (all women) decided to train for and run the United Bank Marathon in Denver in May, 1978, I declined to join them. My self-esteem was still rather low, and I ran for the reason that I knew I *should,* not because it made me feel so good.

Because there aren't too many over-40 runners in our city, I found myself collecting medals and trophies, and this encouraged me to run a bit faster and longer. When you have *never* competed in your life, and therefore *never* won anything, this is a heady feeling. In 1979, I succumbed to the lure of the marathon, and ran in two. In May, I finished the United Bank Marathon in Denver in 4:13 and won first place in age group 40-44. In October I ran the Denver Post Marathon in 3:50, coming in 4th in my age group. My training for both marathons peaked at about 50-55 miles a week. Being a housewife made it easier to schedule training runs, but I know many women who work outside the home, manage families, and *also* run in marathons. They have my respect and admiration.

Following the two marathons in 1979, I was on such an emotional high that I felt compelled to share all this "good stuff" I had found in long-distance running. Advertising for an all-woman Saturday morning fun run brought out 40 women, and from this group a women's running club was developed. Planning meetings, lining up speakers, putting out a monthly newsletter and just talking a lot to beginners has been a wonderful outlet for my energy and enthusiasm for running. I have been so blessed by knowing these women, and I have also been blessed by running itself. My fervor has become almost evangelical in urging people to take care of their bodies. I do not urge everyone to race marathons; rather, to just get out regularly and do something, be it walking, running, bicycling, or swimming.

The impact of running on my diet has been favorable. I am much more conscious of eating a balanced diet. While we still eat meat, there is more fish and poultry included than before, and many new vegetables and fruits. Running has brought about a fondness for beer, but less interest in hard liquor. I never have smoked, and now am vehement in opposing it. I find it difficult to be around smokers for any length of time and resent their every puff. Returning to diet considerations, I find that my weight has remained around 112 (I am 5'2"), perhaps a bit lower just before a marathon, and a bit higher during recovery. For two weeks or so, I just can't seem to get enough to eat! I am much more conscious of what is contained in what I eat, and though I indulge in candy bars, etc., I can keep it at a minimum. We no longer have cookies around the house, and desserts are served only once a week or so. We have switched to whole-wheat bread, and eat more rice than before. I usually have rice or potatoes with every dinner, two vegetables, and often two salads. I use much less of the prepared foods, and do more steaming and baking than frying. I think all of these changes have been a direct result in our whole household becoming more conscious of good health habits.

As to stress management, I believe running has helped me to cope much better with daily problems and tensions. I run alone a lot, and find that a solution to a problem will come during or shortly after a run, even though I do not usually concentrate on solving problems as I run. Some critics might say that I just have fewer stresses than others, because the children are older, etc., but I feel that regardless of my particular stresses, running makes me respond more positively to everything in my life. The depression I experienced a few years ago probably would have been cured by the professional help and medication alone, along with family support; but I feel the running made such a positive contribution to my sense of self-esteem, a feeling I was not well-acquainted with before. Also, running has provided me with a social outlet which was missing in my life. Our family lifestyle has not changed; we are home-oriented and I do not wish to change that. However, the circle of friends I have developed through running, as well as the larger group in the running club, has given my outgoing personality a chance to express itself in a constructive and helpful way.

Much has been written about addiction to running, and I am frequently asked about this by beginning runners. I can definitely say that I *am* addicted to running. The first time I got the flu while training for the 1979 spring marathon, I was devastated, depressed, cried a lot and was very miserable. Much the same reaction followed my first running injury. Now, however, I find a layoff tolerable; I have learned *patience*. When a cold, company, or other circumstances force a layoff, I am patient because I know I will run again, and run well. What I am inside has been given to me in part by running; but what I am inside will not end when the running does . . . .

One final thought (parting shot) . . . George Sheehan has compared running a marathon to giving birth. When I first read that, my reaction was, "How does he know?" . . . But after running three marathons, and having four children, I can say there is definitely a parallel. There is pain, but much joy and pride follow that pain. Not all children "turn out" perfectly, neither do all marathons, but each one has something special to give us, and helps us learn some lessons. I am much like Dr. Sheehan — I could talk about running forever, and so I will close.

That letter was written to me last year by Judy Tucker of Pueblo, Colorado. I am grateful to her for allowing me to share her experience with you.

I'll end this Day's commentary with a passage written decades ago by the late Walter Lippmann. When you finish this reading, take a deep breath, give thanks for all your good fortunes, and enter another dashing check for Day Thirteen. You have entertained the notion of a heroic act — and that is more than most ever have a chance to do.

The best things of mankind are as useless as Amelia Earhart's adventure. In such persons mankind overcomes the inertia which would keep it earthbound forever in its habitual ways. They have in them the free and useless energy with which alone men surpass themselves.

Such energy cannot be planned and managed. It is wild and free. But all the heroes, the saints and the seers, the explorers and the creators, partake of it. They do not know where their impulse is taking them. They have been possessed for a time with an extraordinary passion which is unintelligible in ordinary human terms.

They do the useless, brave, noble, the divinely foolish and the very wisest things that are done by men. And what they prove to themselves and to others is that man is no mere automaton in his routine, no mere cog in the collective machine, but that in the dust of which he is made there is also fire, lighted now and then by great winds from the sky.

— Walter Lippmann

If we could see ourselves as others see us, we may never speak to them again.

— Anonymous

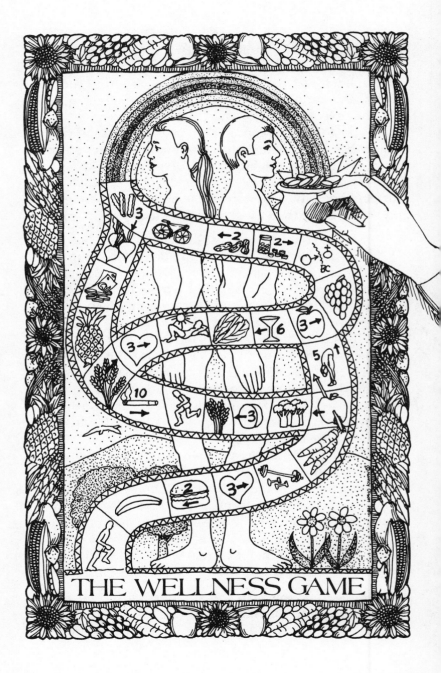

THE WELLNESS GAME

Day Fourteen

Develop And Begin To Carry Out A Personal Wellness Plan

Purpose: To integrate your knowledge about, and interest in, the wellness concept into a systematic personal program which will facilitate the achievement and the enjoyment of your highest and best purposes.

The objective today is to start you on a wellness program for the coming six months. This Day is intended to help you tie it all together — to go to the bank, in effect, with your "winnings" over the past two weeks while playing the Wellness Game.

PERSONAL WELLNESS PLANNING

A plan is a simple, essential, and invaluable tool for wellness. There is nothing mysterious, boring, or complicated about it. A planner is one who *systematically* develops and allocates resources for *optimal* future outcomes. A wellness planner systematically organizes his or her life in order to achieve his/her highest level of total health. I want you to become a planner — specifically, a personal wellness planner. Starting now.

Everybody plans, in one way or another. The difference between what usually occurs and planning for wellness is tied to the italicized terms in the above definition of a planner.

"Systematic" means a group of interrelated elements forming a collective unity, a network of ideas, principles, rules, procedures, etc., a state or condition of harmonious, orderly interaction. "Optimum" means the best or most favorable condition for a particular situation (*American Heritage Dictionary*). You get the idea — a personal wellness plan is a deliberate program for achieving whole-person excellence — the single most favorable level of health status that can be achieved.

There are several reasons why a personal wellness plan is the best available tool for shaping a wellness lifestyle. Let me highlight eight factors which partially explain my enthusiasm for this method of organizing good intentions:

1. Your resources are limited. It makes good sense to husband or expend wisely your limited supply of *time* — you have only so much. In order to build skills, develop capabilities, create options, and enjoy the effects of your human and other investments, you must use time wisely. This is a basic function of a plan.

2. A plan reinforces self-responsibility. At subconscious as well as overt levels, you get to acknowledge that it is your initiative and your follow-through that sets and accomplishes your goals.

3. A plan defines your commitment and intentions. The act of writing down a resolution creates a stronger belief that this is the real thing, that what you are doing is for keeps. It also clarifies your choices. Thus, a plan increases the prospects for goal achievement.

4. You become the cause, rather than the effect, of actions and other variables impacting on your lifestyle.

5. A plan builds confidence and raises self-esteem. For

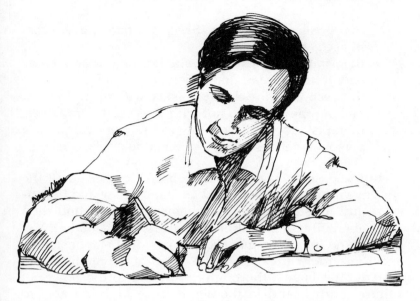

the reasons already noted, you come to acknowledge your-self for the kind of choices being made, and for having the mental strength to see them through.

6. A plan bridges individual action and collective realities. You automatically attend to the norms of disparate cultures in the context of planning processes. This, in turn, advances your odds for personal success and for being able to influence others through your example.

7. A plan facilitates creativity and personal insights. You think more about life purposes and directions. Thus, you experience what some philosophers have termed the "examined life."

8. A plan helps you to take change seriously. When psychologists and others describe the considerations that must be attended if behavior-change intentions are to suc-ceed over time, isolated factors that are a standard part of the plan process are described. These include:

- anticipating that, at first, change will not be easy;
- that immediate action is advisable;

- that goals must be specific, quantifiable, and time-phased;
- that initial expectations should be moderate, as should the pace of first action steps; and
- that responsibility clearly must be with the individual making the changes, not with the parent, employer, therapist, doctor, coach, or guru. (No one can write a personal wellness plan for someone else!)

In the past 13 Days, you have been exposed to all the objective information you need to shape a new and healthier reality. To summarize, you know the basics and then some about fitness, nutrition, and stress management. You understand the preeminent role of personal responsibility, and the minor influence of the "health" or medical care system. You have a thorough grounding in the power of cultural norms, and in the significance of being able to recognize and reshape those values and expectations which do not support and reinforce wellness attitudes and behaviors. You are aware of what it means to be a healthy person beyond just not being sick. And, finally, the idea of going to "heroic" lengths to experience some special quest that complements wellness is not viewed as quite so extreme as it once may have been. Now, it remains only to tie all this knowledge, awareness, and motivation into a plan that insures your best results. Information is one thing; only action will free you from mediocrity, an illness culture, "normal" health, and slow ruin — and set you on your own special path to excellence.

The personal wellness plan is not, of course, the only model for lifestyle change. It is simply the least understood or employed approach. Other change models that get all the attention are: (1) no model at all — many people never make lifestyle changes; (2) the bootstraps model, also known as the Horatio Alger "I did it on my own" approach; (3) the crisis or catastrophe model — heart attacks, earthquakes, plagues, and the like make this "teachable moment" technique very dramatic and expensive; and (4) the serendipity model, which requires that you be in the right place at a terrific time in order that change can come to you. This is the easiest method — if you are very lucky. Unfortunately, you cannot count on it.

THE STEPS IN PERSONAL WELLNESS PLANNING

Developing and carrying out a plan is an enjoyable and challenging process. It is possible to make anything seem complicated, but try not to let it happen to your wellness plan. There are but ten parts to the activity, and you do not have to memorize or spend a great amount of time learning to master any one of them. Here, simply stated, are the basic steps in personal wellness planning.

1. Select a life area for development in the plan. Depending on how you like to organize things, there could be 6-60 life areas for which to plan. I think everything can be included in about six life areas, those being:

- optimal health
- business/profession
- money/financial security
- self-development
- having fun
- primary relationships/family

In beginning your personal wellness plan for the six months to come, I recommend that you begin with the life area of optimal health, since these considerations and possibilities are fresh in your mind from the readings over the past 13 Days.

2. Generate a clarity about your life purposes. Having a clear sense of direction in life is not something that comes automatically or easily to most people. Think of

.some of the most fundamental questions, and ask yourself where you stand on the issues, how you got to these beliefs, and how committed you are to their realization. Here are a few samplers:

- Who has had the greatest influence on your current value system?
- How close are your values and those of your parents?
- What is your most important reason for living?
- What are at least five other purposes for your existence?
- If you had a week to live, what would you do with your time?
- Are you having enough fun in life?
- What would you like that you do not now have?
- Who is a part of your life that you could do nicely without?
- Who is not a part of your life that should be?

These are just examples of the kinds of questions you can generate to discover your current purposes in order to fashion modifications, if necessary. Some believe that our purposes change as we think more intensively about them; others suggest that we simply become aware of purposes we had all along but did not recognize.

In either case, a consideration of purposes is essential to the next step in personal wellness planning, namely, defining goals.

3. Identify wellness goals and objectives. All the steps in the personal-wellness-plan process are not equal in significance. All are valuable, all are helpful, and all deserve the modest time involved to carry them out. None, however, is as important as the goal-setting stage. Give this activity your best effort. Goals should be specific and measurable. Nothing complicated about that. Instead of a goal that reads: "To lose weight," the goal would be "To lose 20 pounds in six months." To help you further understand

and commit yourself to the goal, follow it with an objective(s). For instance, an objective might be: "I want to achieve this goal in order to feel good about wearing a trendy bathing suit at the pool." (There is no law requiring that all goals and objectives be designed to make the world a safer place.) Or, see if you can develop positive goals for whichever life area is being planned. Another optimal health goal, positively phrased, might be, "To develop a capacity to utilize three stress-management techniques by the time of my next birthdate." The objective or rationale for this goal might be related to your desire to become more effective in difficult situations, to preserve your energies, and to assist others by your example.

It might be a good idea to start your personal wellness planning in the optimal health area with at least one goal addressed to a desired outcome in each of the five wellness dimensions.

4. List a number of goal-supportive actions. In other words, what specific actions will you take, or commit to beginning now, to advance toward the realization of your goals? List at least three initiatives you will act upon today, or in the coming days and weeks, to solidify and make real your goals, and set you on a path leading to their realization. If your goal is to be able to swim a mile in 20 minutes by the time of the next reunion of your high school swim team, goal-supportive activity statements might include:

- buy a six-month membership in the local swim club so I have access to the pool and the support of others who can give encouragement and a little coaching.
- buy a swim suit, ear plugs, and goggles — tomorrow.
- rearrange my schedule so that nothing else will be in competition for my time during the selected part of the day.

5. Identify the barriers that will or might get in the way. One day, you write a set of goals and resolve to move mountains to achieve them. But, if you forget to identify *which* mountains have to be moved, or circumvented, you could get blocked the next day, or within the next week or two. Listing barriers between you and goal achievement serves to bring hazards and difficulties ahead into conscious awareness, and allows you time to ponder alternate strategies for dealing with such obstacles. The operating principle here is not unlike preparing for any event: practice, anticipation, and planning lead to improved performance.

There are two parts to barrier identification in personal wellness planning. The first is to write all the reasons why the goal will or might not be achievable. For instance, if your goal were to gradually shift toward a food pattern characteristic of optimal-performance dining by Thanksgiving Day, the barriers might be:

- My husband likes steak and potatoes four times a week.
- Food habits are impossible to change — I cannot give up Twinkies.
- The children will never go along.
- The crowd at the office will think I'm some kind of health nut.
- It will be too expensive.
- Aunt Fanny's feelings will be hurt if I don't eat her chocolate glumps.
- It will be too much trouble.
- I do not know a soul who dines the way I want to for optimal living.
- I don't know how to do it.

The second step is to write, after each barrier, how you intend to deal with it. Be realistic. Pretend for a moment that the above list of barriers was indeed your own for this particular goal; then write a line or two describing how you would deal with each of these obstacles.

6. Identify the nature of payoffs and visualize yourself enjoying the realization of your goals. You can strengthen your enthusiasm and extend the depth of your commitment to the goals selected by clarifying, dwelling upon, even fantasizing about the delights associated with their achievement. Doing so further moves the process into conscious awareness, and thereby enhances your desire, even lust, for goal accomplishment.

Here is an example of how this step works. Suppose your goal was to hike from one end of the John Muir Trail to the other in not more than 30 days this coming summer. Every night, before retiring, you would employ the visualization skills you started practicing during Day 11, in order to see yourself successfully negotiating the spectacular trails as the days of summer pass by. You would give special attention to the celebration that awaits you at the conclusion of your quest, and note the tremendous feelings of pride and accomplishment you attach to the realization of this noble goal. (You could have almost as much fun thinking about this endeavor as doing it! And, you would not exhaust yourself or have to worry about bears, poison oak, or mosquitoes.) Other goal payoffs to think about might include reflections on:

- How terrific you look.
- The extraordinary amount of energy you have at work and after work.
- How satisfying it is to be responsible for your health and success.
- How wildly popular you have become, even though you do not need approval from others in order to feel good about yourself.
- The pleasures involved in being so romantic and hip, sexy and free.
- The joys of being tax-exempt and able to get better gas mileage because of your wellness lifestyle!

7. Design a set of supportive environments. Improve the odds for plan implementation. Set it up so your goal pursuits do not become heroic acts, unless that is your objective. Think about the people around you at work who might want to join you in the Wellness Game. Do the same for the home situation, and among your friends. Even if others do not want to bother, at least work with them so they do not get in the way. Consider the kind of norm changes that would make your goal pursuits easier in many of the most influential cultures in which you find yourself. For example, if you have a goal of establishing a wellness program at your place of business that involves 20% of the work force within the first year of operation, you obviously must involve a lot of others. You will, early on, figure out that certain job norms get in the way (e.g., the "hurry-up" periods every three hours, the vending machine contents, the spy system, the high-decibel levels, and the fact that 80 percent of the employees chain-smoke cheap cigars!). Thus, support-group formation, training, and guidance will come naturally. However, even for personal goals that do not directly involve others (e.g., to bike ten miles a day for one entire month), a support system is a big help. Using the just-noted goal example, the support phase of your personal wellness plan might find you writing down elements such as:

- To have Jane, Ira, and _____ride with me on specific days of the week.
- To have my boyfriend, my sister, and my father-in-law ask me every afternoon if I completed my ride yet.
- To have Horace prepare delicious and nutritious smoothies to hand to me upon my return from each day's ride.
- To have my friend Hortense take my picture on the 30th day as I complete my ride — and achieve my goal.

You get the idea. Remember to write down the details about your support system intentions. If possible, have others agree, in writing, to assist you in the achievement of your wellness plan.

8. Keep a log or notebook to record successes, feelings, thoughts, crises, and so on. In a sense, a log is a safe place to centralize your memoirs. This can later prove insightful, enjoyable, and satisfying. A log, however, is also valuable for another reason: It solidifies and strengthens dedication to your wellness goals. You see, every time you open the log — a record of what you have already invested in pursuing wellness goals — you are reminded, as well, of the action steps for goal achievement to which you have made a personal commitment.

A log is a private record of your reactions along the way. It is best kept *for your eyes only.* Share your goals, if you wish; publish your plan in the *Wall Street Journal* or a lonely-hearts-club magazine. But keep your log strictly for your private collection. In this way, you will be more likely to record *all* matters and thoughts of consequence.

9. Develop a set of bench marks or measures that tell you how you are doing. When you look over the goals you have identified, figure out a way to progress from where you are to where you want to be in three months, a year, or whenever. Then, plot a set of bench marks, measures, watershed indicators, or whatever you choose to call the periods or stages along the way. These too, like the log, will reinforce your intentions as you move along. They will also provide objective feedback about how things are going.

An example may be in order. Suppose one of your wellness goals was "To learn to play the flute in time to play a solo piece at the next family reunion a year from now — at a level of competence wherein they and I enjoy the performance." Surely you do not want to wait a year to assess how well you are doing. Bench marks might be set at every quarter; you could arrange feedback from music teachers, recital audiences, friends, other flute players, and so on. You may find, after a few bench mark periods, that this goal is "in the bag." Thus, you can select a more demanding piece to play at the reunion. Or, forget the reunion — play at the Lincoln Center in New York with the Metropolitan Opera.

10. Evaluate the plan. Both during and at the conclusion of the planning period, assessments are in order. In the first case, be alert to whether the goal is still as valued as in the beginning, whether it was too easy or too difficult. In the latter case (end of plan period), ask yourself if the goal provided the kinds of payoffs you anticipated. If not, what would?

The key consideration about evaluation is to insure that the plan is serving you, not the reverse. The satisfactions you derive from a conscious, systematic approach to your highest potential are vastly more important than the vehicle you select to get you there.

Evaluation is a double-edged sword: it can work for or against you. The latter might apply if, every time the going gets rough, you look up at the obstacles and barriers and say to yourself: "Hey man, this calls for evaluation," and proceed to set lesser goals. Have scheduled times for evaluation of goals; once a month might do quite nicely. At other times, the goals are not to be tampered with or reconsidered.

SUMMARY

The personal wellness plan is the culmination of the 14-Day program for wellness. It will be the centerpiece of your efforts to establish a lifelong quest for whole-person excellence.

The plan can be written on the back of an envelope (you have to write *very* small or have a huge envelope), in a bound hard-cover book with gold-leaf trim, or something in between. Just put it in writing and work with it as often as you can, preferably daily.

Write a contract with yourself to fulfill the terms and conditions of the plan. Have it witnessed by friends, a mate, or members of the support group that will assist you in the pursuit of one or more goals.

Think of the personal wellness plan as part of the equipment that makes it easier to play, enjoy, and win at the Wellness Game.

Think of it as your map to a wellness path that only you can discover — and explore — in this lifetime.

You now have all the data you need to make it happen. You have *done* what is necessary to *do* it — to live a wellness lifestyle. For further encouragement, information, and inspiration, read about what some are doing on an institutional level to make it easier for others to join in bringing about or, more accurately, speeding up, the wellness revolution.

This is your last flourishing check on the 14-Day calendar. Make it a good one.

Part Two

Wellness Innovations:
A Sampling of
Creative Programs

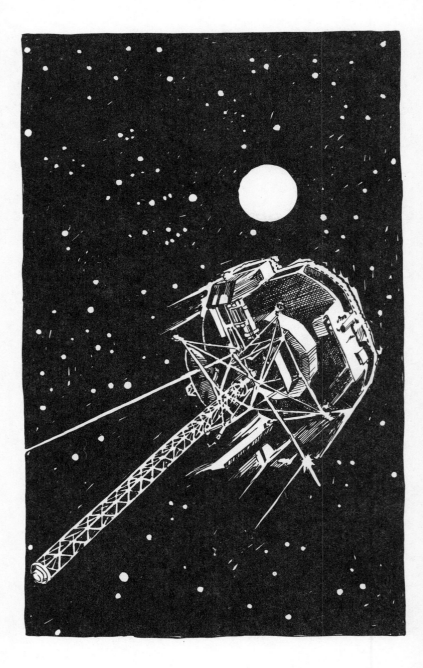

Part Two

Wellness Innovations:
A Sampling of
Creative Programs

Wellness has, in recent years, moved toward becoming a part of mainstream North American culture. The reasons for this rapid recognition and growing popularity are varied. Among the factors most often cited are: frustration with rising medical system costs; the fact that awesome technologies and treatment breakthroughs do not seem to advance health status; a rising consciousness about the merits and satisfactions of physical fitness; the parallel growth of "holistic" forms of participant-centered caring; and the increasing support for a shift in perception that health is an individual rather than a medical or governmental responsibility. Connected with this last point is an unchallenged awareness that what people do or do not do for themselves regarding habits, behaviors and attitudes has more effect on health status than the quality or availability of doctors, hospitals, drugs, and medical programs. No doubt these and other conditions are and have been influential, directly and indirectly, in the rising popularity of wellness as a desirable lifestyle approach to the pursuit of best potentials for physical, psychological, and spiritual well-being.

However, all these factors put together are not as significant, in my view, as the roles played by leading individual and institutional innovators.

This section briefly highlights the range and extent of wellness programs throughout the U.S. and Canada. The listing of innovators is illustrative, rather than complete. Further, the program descriptions are not intended to be detailed or totally current. (Almost by definition, innovators keep innovating, so the forms, numbers and details keep changing.)

What you should obtain from this vignette is a sense for the richness, depth, and creativity that marks the wellness revolution to date.

If you are in a position to influence a school, hospital, corporation, or other institution toward wellness programming in the years to come, perhaps the following account will also provide a few hints to speed you along. The primary reason these institutions have gone so far is not a condition of their wealth, power, or superior virtue. Instead, it is because one or more wellness-oriented individuals within or connected with the organization took risks at opportune moments and made the necessary commitments and agreements that led to change and innovation.

Thus, what follows is both an abbreviated overview and an acknowledgment tribute to a number of creative individuals. Their influence and judgment have made the wellness concept a reality as well as a theory. Because of their influence, a wellness lifestyle in years ahead is more likely to become a logical choice, rather than a heroic act. That is why this book is dedicated to these innovators, and why I am grateful for having had opportunities to work with them, or otherwise learn about their beginnings.

Feel free to write, visit, call, or otherwise check out in more detail any or all of the programs mentioned. Addresses and phone numbers are provided; inquiries are welcomed.

To the innovative institutions — congratulations and Godspeed for continued success. To the innovators themselves — good wishes, be well, and many thanks.

HOSPITALS AS FUTURE HOUSES OF WELL REPUTE*

In early 1974, a Mill Valley, California, physician named John

---

*A portion of this account was first published in *Medical Self Care Magazine,* Summer 1981, pp. 30-31.

Travis hung a shingle outside his office declaring it a "Wellness Resource Center." Travis said he would see no sick people, prescribe no pills, treat no illnesses, nor wear a white coat. Instead, this self-styled "doctor of well-being" would work with client-participants who wanted to learn how to become healthier, not only for illness avoidance but also for the personal enrichment inherent in physical and mental "superhealth."

The conventional wisdom was that Travis' health-promotion practice might be a hit in trendy, affluent Marin County, where Mill Valley is located, but not in the real world, where people have enough trouble paying for sickness care to think about getting healthier for its own sake.

It's seven years later now, and the conventional wisdom was wrong on two counts. Travis' Wellness Resource Center never really made it in Marin County,* but wellness as a social movement has grown to dramatic proportions throughout the United States and Canada. Wellness is big all over: in many corporations, physicians' offices, schools, public agencies, private organizations — and surprisingly, in hospitals.

If anyone had asked Travis or other wellness pioneers if hospitals might become influential in popularizing the concept, they would have replied, "Unlikely." But the fact is, hospitals have taken a leading role in the wellness revolution.

WHY HOSPITALS?

Wellness programs have flourished in hospitals for at least five reasons. Some of them may not be universally considered the "right" motivations — that is, "pure" and noble in purpose — but that should be of little concern. My own view is that the right thing done for the wrong reasons is *still* the right thing.

· To a certain extent, hospitals got involved in wellness because it was great public relations. Administrators and trustees

---

*Of course, hospitals and others in the heartlands beyond Mill Valley would be hard pressed to succeed if they were not favored with financial backing during the start-up period. The fact is that Travis never did have financial assistance from any foundation, insurance fund, government grant, or private donor, as do almost all the current centers. Thus, the critical variable for "success" may be more a condition of financial heritage than geographical position.

discovered that their institutions could garner as much favorable media attention for dedicating $100,000 health-enrichment centers as they could for dedicating new wings for space-age medical care that cost millions.

· Another motivation was to improve the health of hospital employees. Increasing employee health-care costs have strained hospital budgets. Administrators hoped that in-house health-promotion activities might slow rising health insurance costs and other illness-related expenditures, for example, the costs involved in training replacements for those who leave their jobs for health reasons.

· A third attraction of health promotion was the prospect of making money, particularly from the sale of "package programs" to local business and industry.

· Another had to do with the personal interests of hospital planning directors, administrators, and trustees.

· Finally, and perhaps the least motivating but clearly the most publicly professed reason for inaugurating hospital wellness centers was the desire to promote public health. Many times hospital charters would be resurrected to show that promoting the health of the community was a cornerstone of the institution's purpose, and that wellness was a return to the hospital's roots. In most hospital wellness programs, these motivating factors have operated to varying degrees.

The word "wellness" is used broadly at most hospitals involved in health promotion, and their programs reflect this loose interpretation. Under the wellness banner, programs range from traditional one-shot patient education projects to comprehensive programs for multidimensional health enrichment. In the former, the goal is to *reduce the risk* of becoming sick. In the latter, the goal is to *promote health-enrichment activities* for the payoffs intrinsic in feeling healthy. The one seeks to minimize losses, the other to maximize gains. In a traditional one-shot program, participants would be encouraged to quit smoking to prevent lung cancer years hence. In a more comprehensive program, that advice would be coupled with jogging training or a swimming class where participants could begin to feel physiological changes in their bodies within a month or two.

A truly comprehensive wellness project would offer programs in all five dimensions.

Today, in this dawning stage of hospital wellness centers, few programs encompass all five dimensions listed above. Why not? Largely because the programs must be economically viable. Hospitals that sponsor wellness centers must meet their costs, otherwise their health promotion endeavors, no matter how well intended, will fail. At present, there is a larger market for relatively inexpensive limited-purpose, short-term wellness activities than there is for more comprehensive wellness programs. Therefore, today's hospital wellness centers tend to offer single-purpose programs in one or more of the five basic areas. Beyond that, they usually encourage participants to expand their wellness interests into some of the other areas as they see their health situations improve. (There are exceptions, as will be noted shortly.)

Comprehensive programs hold tremendous promise for the future, but until more people learn that they can win at the Wellness Game, until their thinking progresses beyond illness prevention to a recognition of the joys of a balanced, healthy lifestyle, hospital wellness programs will have to recruit participants by focusing on specific, largely single-issue needs such as stop-smoking courses, obesity clinics, or cooking classes for diabetics.

A DOCTOR IN THE HOUSE OF WELL REPUTE? PROBABLY NOT

Despite the fact that hospitals have long been doctor-workshops, physicians have played only minor roles in the hospital-based wellness movement. The doctors' major contribution thus far has been not to get in the way. Naturally, a few fitness-oriented holistically inclined M.D.s strategically situated in hospital hierarchies have been instrumental in launching some hospital-based wellness centers, but this has been the exception rather than the rule.

Hospital wellness advocates have developed the following strategy for integrating wellness facilities into their institutions. They have solicited doctors' advice, invited doctor participation, and kept physicians fully informed of wellness center activities. They have avoided linking "wellness" to "holistic health," because the unorthodox treatments used in some holistic healing arts generate anxiety and opposition among doctors. Hospital wellness advocates have also learned not to knock medicine to promote wellness. So far this strategy has worked.

PATIENTS LAST

Hospitals with wellness programs generally offer them to everyone within range of their facilities — except hospital patients. Hospital employees are usually the first wellness center client group. They may be offered incentives to participate, such as cash bonuses, time off, or other inducements. Next come community residents, usually on a walk-in basis. Finally, the wellness center reaches out to specific target groups — industry, business or professional groups.

So far, however, hospital-based wellness facilities have not reached out to hospital patients. There are several reasons for this. One is that it's safer to develop and test new health programs on relatively healthy people just in case mistakes are made. Another is to maintain doctors' support. It's one thing for the medical community to tolerate strange goings-on in distant hospital outposts; it's quite another to have wellness promoters messing around with sick patients. Of course, if wellness if to fulfill its promise to seize the "teachable moment" and interest patients in lifestyle change when they tend to be most open to it, then this situation will have to change. For the present, however, hospital wellness center staff are nearly unanimous in the opinion that patients will be incorporated into their activities in the future, when health-enrichment programs have become more sophisticated, and when the political climate permits.

THE LARGER QUESTION

Hospitals may be jumping on the wellness bandwagon, but a larger question remains: Why go to a hospital for wellness? Can't most people get involved in wellness activities on their own? Just about everyone who practices a wellness lifestyle found his or her unique path without help from hospital-based wellness centers or, for that matter, from schools, employers, free-standing centers or anyone else.

The real issue, however, is not whether people *need* hospital-based wellness centers, but whether such facilities *help*. Do they contribute to the likelihood that more people will learn about, choose and then maintain health-enriching activities and healthier lifestyles? I would say "yes."

Norman Cousins, in his popular book *Anatomy of an Illness*, states that hospitals are no place for sick people! Perhaps this reputation will improve as the wellness movement takes hold in thousands of hospitals in the years to come. Perhaps hospitals will no longer be just hospitals ministering to disease and disaster cases, but will also become centers for higher education in whole-person well-being. When this occurs, every area will be proud to have in its midst a house of well repute.

In the following section, you will read about some concrete actions being taken by the leading wellness-oriented hospitals, beginning with the work of the American Hospital Association's support for and commitment to this idea.

CENTER FOR HEALTH PROMOTION OF THE AMERICAN HOSPITAL ASSOCIATION

A lot of the credit for the activities of hospitals currently operating wellness programs is due to the leadership of the AHA's Center for Health Promotion. Established by the AHA in 1978 for the purpose of encouraging and providing assistance to hospitals in health promotion, the Center has progressed beyond the expectations of its most ardent supporters.

In just a few years, the Center has rapidly expanded in staff size, responsibilities, scope of work, and influence within the overall AHA system. The major reason for this is that the Center staff is providing a complex of services and benefits to member hospitals in wellness and related health-promotion areas that are highly valued at the present time.

The Center has contributed to the growth of the wellness movement in general by sponsoring national seminars on health promotion, commissioning papers on specific issues, conducting surveys, and providing resource people as consultants to institutions requiring special assistance. The Center also publishes a regular health promotion newsletter, is a good source for telephone consultations on hospital-related wellness developments, and has produced audio-visual packages for health promotion purposes.

However, if ever there were a contest to find the single event that did the most to advance the state of the art, I think the Center would be competitive on the basis of its role in sponsoring the annual "Innovator's Conference." At these spring affairs, usually held at AHA Headquarters in Chicago, teams of selected administrators, physicians, planners, and other professionals who play the key roles in the most advanced hospital-based wellness and other health promotion programs are involved in two-and-a-half day intensives. The sessions are set up to insure the widest possible sharing of knowledge and the wisdom of common experience with comparable challenges and opportunities. The Innovator Conferences are strictly invitational: it is not who you know so much as what you have done that gets a hospital an invitation to send a team to these sessions. While a number of outside experts are brought in to address the future of wellness and other types of issues, and to stimulate the attendees to consider expanded possibilities, most of the time is given to working sessions on issues such as marketing, physician involvement, the use of advanced media techniques, coordination with local resource people, and so on. The meetings serve a twin purpose: they enable the innovators to meet each other, share observations, and avoid reinventing the wellness wheel. In addition, they provide a wealth of solid information for hospitals just getting started in health promotion and desirous of knowing what has worked (and what has not).

The administrators at AHA deserve a lot of credit for having the foresight in 1978 to know that a constituency for health promotion would emerge from the hospital community they serve. However, the special vote from this corner for distinguished service to the cause goes to the staff members of the Center for the roles they have played in working within the system, selecting the right issues, the proper people, and the best times to move to the next step.

Every institutional grouping (i.e., schools, business, and so on) should have a Center for Health Promotion looking out for and otherwise stimulating and serving them.

For information contact:

Mary Longe, Staff Specialist
Center for Health Promotion
American Hospital Association

840 North Lake Shore Drive
Chicago, Illinois 60611
(312) 280-6048

INNOVATIVE HOSPITAL-BASED WELLNESS CENTERS

The AHA's Center for Health Promotion counts thirty-some hospitals as innovators for the purpose of invitations to the annual conferences. In fact, there are closer to 100 deserving hospitals (as of late 1981) which could be included if space and logistics were suitable. To offer a sense for the range of activity, I've included brief vignettes about wellness programming at the hospitals which I know best.

Let us begin this little tour in Indianapolis.

ST. VINCENT HOSPITAL AND HEALTH CARE CENTER

St. Vincent Hospital and Health Care Center is a not-for-profit organization established in 1881 by the Daughters of Charity of St. Vincent de Paul. The corporate symbol of St. Vincent Hospital and Health Care Center is three doves in flight. The doves, as signs of peace and life, are a trio representing the hospital's attention to the needs of the body, mind, and soul of each patient. Flying in concord, the doves symbolize outreach to meet growing health needs of the community. The Wellness Center is just one of the ways St. Vincent Hospital and Health Care Center serves the community.

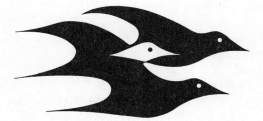

The wellness program is located in a shopping center about nine miles from the hospital and health care center. It has been in operation less than two years as of this writing, but has already introduced tens of thousands of "Hoosiers" to wellness through its quarterly newsletters, seminars, TV programs, wellness fairs, and class offerings. The Center itself is the focus of the program which has outreach to other than the "true believers" as one of its major objectives. Often, unwary shoppers are lured by curiosity to investigate the goings-on in the little building (rumored to have been a teenage disco under previous management) of 8900 square feet in the middle of the Mohawk Place shopping area. Once inside, hapless little old ladies (some in tennis shoes), macho truck drivers, chain-smoking hard-hatters, and bored, Junior League dropouts, suddenly find themselves completely exposed to a new kind of lifestyle called *very* high level wellness. Fortunately, the range of choices is so extensive (over 30 different courses and seminars) that 5,300 people signed on during the first year of wellness at St. Vincent. A major effort toward wellness-lifestyle assessment and change was recently completed with the personnel of a local fire department.

Present plans are ambitious: a series of videotapes on various wellness themes are in preparation; policy changes are being promoted through the offices of sympathetic congressmen (focused on incentives for the adoption of personal responsibility); a wellness-based, employee-assistance program is being developed for the 2,800 employees of the hospital; long-term, health promotion affiliations are being created with two national companies; and two national conferences on the wellness concept are set for the coming months. In addition, memberships in the Center are now available which entitle subscribers to discounts on lectures, classes, events, and resource directories. For For more information about wellness at St. Vincent check with:

Barbara Burke, Assistant Manager HRD
St. Vincent Wellness Center
622 South Range Line Road
Carmel, Indiana 46032
(317) 846-7037

RIVERSIDE HOSPITAL

Located in Toledo, Ohio, Riverside is in the wellness business because of the strong commitment of President Erie Chapman III, and the Riverside Hospital Board of Directors, to wellness as a fundamental responsibility of a community-oriented hospital. A professional staff of six, recruited on a national basis, manages the operation. The hospital board of directors drafted a resolution in support of the project, and the foundation committee has committed $300,000 of hospital memorial trust funds to cover expenses incurred in the initial years of the center's operation. A certificate-of-need proposal for the project was approved by health planning agencies at the regional and state levels, and the hospital has received a commendation from the Northwest Ohio Health Planning Agency for its innovative project.

A team approach, using management by objectives techniques, has been applied to the five wellness dimensions. Special attention is being given to linking wellness programs for employees and their families to future packages marketable to industry and other individuals and groups from the community.

Riverside is paying particular attention to new methods of attracting broad-based participation. For example, consideration is being given to the use of the techniques and methodology of political campaigns as a vehicle for expanding participation in the program.

Riverside is playing a major role in supporting neighborhood revitalization, including renovation of hundreds of housing units and addressing critical public issues that affect health at the lower rungs of Maslow's heirarchy. The developing wellness center blends nicely with these important long-range commitments and should make wellness more acceptable to the diverse groups included in the Riverside constituency.

An active employee advisory committee is helping the staff to spread the program throughout the institution. Renovation and expansion of an older unused building on the hospital campus will soon provide a 29,000-square-foot wellness center (at a cost of over $2 million) connected to the hospital and housing exercise areas and equipment, a resource and learning center, teaching classrooms, an instructional kitchen, a participant evaluation area, a sixteenth-of-a-mile indoor running track, and shower and changing facilities (California hot tub and sauna included). Some who keep watch on such things are looking to Riverside as the hospital most likely to break new ground in wellness initiatives in the years to come.

For more information about Riverside, contact:

George Randt, M.D.
Director, Center for Health Promotion
(419) 726-9552, or
Vice President, Administrative Services
(419) 729-5151 Ext. 343
Riverside Hospital
1600 N. Superior
Toledo, Ohio 43604

SWEDISH WELLNESS SYSTEMS, INC.

Located in Englewood, Colorado, Swedish Medical Center's wellness program is distinguished for several reasons, not the least of which is that it was the first hospital to enter the wellness business. As usual, this happened because a few people were committed to wellness ideals well before the movement was underway or had received unofficial sanctioning from various medical authorities. Principal among them are Winston Howard, former chairman of the Medical Center Board and current chairman of the Wellness Corporation Board, and John Oswald, the current senior vice-president of operations of the Medical Center. Long before the American Hospital Association set up the Center for Health Promotion (noted above), SWC was serving as a resource center for the rest of the institutions wanting to know how to get started. For playing this role with generosity and skill, SWC will always deserve a special place in the ranks of wellness promoters.

From the beginning, SWC has seen its role as a catalytic and coordinative one. By involving professionals in the various dimensions of wellness from throughout the community, SWC has developed a diverse and well-integrated program that far exceeds what could have been accomplished on its own. There is at present a community resource base of over 100 professionals and organizations that are used in SWC programs on a brokerage basis; the budget for wellness is over a half-million dollars per year; and eleven full-time professionals serve hospital, employee, industry, school, and community client groups.

Because of its community and resource development approach, it should come as no surprise to learn that SWC has joined with Dr. Robert Allen and the Human Resources Institute (discussed elsewhere) in advocating and further developing the Lifegain culture change system. The combining of efforts of these prominent forces in wellness promises to produce major new initiatives in the field for years to come.

Two of the most recent innovations to come out of this joint effort are an office-based physicians' wellness program and a national network of hospitals. Both of these use the Lifegain system and are intended to further integrate the medical care system into the wellness movement. The hospital network is particularly exciting because it provides hospitals interested in wellness the opportunity to take advantage of the program development that has been done by SWC and HRI, and to be a part of a national wellness delivery system. The potential impact of these synergistic efforts of hospitals throughout the country is enormous.

Finally, SWC continues to design and sponsor national conferences in the Rocky Mountains for hospitals and other organizations from throughout North America. These conferences provide information on the innovative and justly famous Swedish Wellness Program for building both internal and external enthusiasm for health-enhancement lifestyles and the capability to sustain them through deliberate culture change.

Swedish Wellness Center is truly a network of people and organizations who believe change is possible.

For more information, write or call:
Bob Gorsky, Director
Swedish Wellness Systems, Inc.
3444 South Emerson Street
Englewood, Colorado 80110
(303) 789-6940

GROWING YOUNGER

Growing Younger is a year-old neighborhood wellness program for persons aged 60 and over in Boise, Idaho. It combines fun and friendships to facilitate culture change for health at the block level. In just over a year, the sponsoring agencies (Healthwise Inc. and the Boise Council on Aging) have enlisted and trained over 850 of the city's eligible population of 20,000 seniors. The goal is to involve ten percent by 1984.

Growing Younger was initially funded in October, 1980, as part of the Centers for Disease Control's Risk Reduction Program. As the only risk reduction program specifically focused on older adults, it has been promoted as a national model for replication in other communities. In 1982, principal funding for Growing Younger was transferred to the State of Idaho through the federal block grant process. State funding for the third year is budgeted at $125 per participant. Participant fees of $8 per person or $10 per couple go directly to offset the cost of materials.

From the beginning, Growing Younger has been warmly received throughout the community. Local corporations, hospitals, public agencies and employee associations have supported the program through donations of cash, materials and printing services which have kept participant fees low and allowed scholarships for those unable to pay.

Growing Younger is designed for replication in a wide variety of communities. A comprehensive replication package including instructors guides, organization plans and promotional materials will be available to potential sponsors.

Inquiries should be addressed to:
Donald W. Kemper
Healthwise, Inc.
Box 1989
Boise, Idaho 83701
(208) 345-1161

FROST VALLEY YMCA

Summer camp is a place to have fun, be outdoors, make new friends, learn fresh skills, and explore exciting places. At its best, this is what camp was about for many of us. In upstate New York, there is a summer camp that offers an added dimension — the opportunity to grow a high level wellness lifestyle.

Since 1978, at least four thousand youngsters from 7 to 18 years of age have been given a variety of opportunities to experience full-scale wellness education as part of a summer vacation. The program is now way beyond the experimental stage, and has in fact become a model emulated by the YMCA and other youth organizations throughout the nation.

The Frost Valley YMCA camp and conference facilities cover 4,500 acres, nestled in the most remote section of 240,000 wilderness acres in the Catskill Mountains. The resident camping program is available for children from every part of the United States and abroad. In addition, Frost Valley runs two- to six-week backpacking, canoeing, and bicycling trips throughout the United States and Canada for teenagers and adults, family camping, conference retreats, cross-country ski outings in winter, and environmental education resident programs during the school year.

Approximately 450 children attend Frost Valley's summer resident camps for each two-week period; allowing for those who stay additional periods, the summer population of campers is about 1,200. Frost Valley has all the usual activities — swimming and boating, tennis, rock climbing and rappeling, gymnastics, basketball, hiking, field sports, campfires, horseback riding, hay rides, trout fishing, assorted "new" games, archery, and so forth. These activities, which provide ample opportunities for fun, outdoor experiences, new friendships and skills, and explorations, are props for the main act: a comprehensive, low-key opportunity for campers to experience all phases of a wellness lifestyle.

A number of factors came together to create the right conditions for wellness to flourish at Frost Valley. There was, as usual, an innovative and supportive board of directors, a cadre of experts willing to devote time to design the program, a capable staff to carry it out, and a population of young innocents who did not really know what they were getting into when they arrived in camp. The success of wellness programming at Frost Valley has been ensured by three additional factors: the stimulation and guidance given by Dr. Bill Hettler as camp physician (see the discussion about wellness at the University of Wisconsin); the energetic role played by D. Halbe Brown, Executive Director of Frost Valley YMCA; and the financial support provided by numerous organizations, such as the Geraldine Dodge Foundation and the Victoria Foundation (the same group that funds the Urban Council on Adolescence and Wellness described elsewhere).

There are many interesting features of the wellness program at Frost Valley. The activities — whether structured or spontaneous — are guided by college-age counselors in the course of regular camp life. Staff members are selected on the basis of their commitment to wellness living and their sensitivity to the needs of youth. Care is given to orient the parents about the nature of wellness as a special feature of camp life. A generous supply of films and books (including numerous wellness activities appearing in a "Counselor Wellness Manual" developed by Frost Valley) are available for use by the staff. Nutritious meals are served in the dining halls, and there are no "junk" food snacks available. In short, the people and environment at Frost Valley are supportive of wellness living.

For more on the details of wellness in a summer camp setting, contact:

Michael Ketcham
Director of Camping
Frost Valley YMCA
Oliverea, New York 12462

Afterword

The director of every program described in this section was given an opportunity to review what I wrote for accuracy. Michael Ketcham of Frost Valley appended a note to the copy, a part of which I thought might be of interest to you:

> We feel flattered to know that you are considering the inclusion of Frost Valley in your book. Progress continues to be made — wellness is an accepted part of camp life (in all that we do); our staff are conscientious and caring individuals who have an interest in interpreting wellness for their campers; and parents are supportive of our programs. In short, while we still have a long way to go, we are getting closer to that "10" you once referred to.

UNIVERSITY OF WISCONSIN HEALTH SERVICE AND LIFESTYLE IMPROVEMENT PROGRAM

The goal at UW-Stevens Point is excellence in health programming to advance the pursuit of wellness. Though students comprise the first target audience, the influence of the program goes beyond Stevens Point, Wisconsin, and even the U.S.

It is hard to abbreviate a report on wellness at this institution. This summary does not dwell on clinical care at the Student Health Service, though 20,000 annual visits might suggest that it is not exactly an afterthought for the staff of 20-some professionals. Nor does this sketch give a sense for the quality and influence of the Lifestyle Assessment Questionnaire, which has had about 60,000 users over the last four years. The focus of this account is on just two of the contributions that the Bill Hettler-led wellness enterprises at UW-SP have made in advancing the movement. These are the annual wellness-promotion-strategies workshops and the promotion of campus wellness by the training and imaginative utilization of student wellness counselors and promoters.

The student program is founded on the idea that improved knowledge, skills, and attitudes require not only intellect but five other dimensions as well: fitness/nutrition, spiritual values, emotional maturity, social/community ties, and occupational/vocational capabilities. The wellness program creates the conditions for the student to learn about, practice, and serve others in all six areas of rounded excellence. A vast range of opportunities is available for students to explore health concerns regarding treatment, illness prevention, and especially the promotion of the wellness ethic. Formal and informal training programs lead to accredited wellness-promotion endeavors throughout the year, such as counseling, presentations at all grade levels, attendance at wellness conferences, development of courses, retreats, personal wellness planning, and so on through a mind-boggling array of choices — to participate fully in shaping what are intended as lifetime super-health patterns. In short, there is a trained army of wellness enthusiasts on the watch for more recruits at UW-SP. (It must be no fun for low-lifers.)

Here is an edited summary of 30 activities of the student wellness teams, as reported in the 1980 Annual Report cited earlier. It lends a measure of specificity to the notion that peer influence can be one very powerful force in affecting both individual behavior and cultural influences.

1. An increase in positive alternatives to vending machines on campus.
2. A list of the caloric content of foods, showing the advantages to alternatives in all food service operations.
3. The provision of additional spaces for quiet time, so individuals have an opportunity for reflection, meditation, and relaxation.
4. Creation of a lifestyle-development lab where individuals

assess themselves and begin to make improvements.

5. Improvements in the food service operation.
6. Advertising to increase the awareness and utilization of wellness offerings on the campus.
7. An increase in nonsmoking areas in academic buildings, residence halls, food service areas, and lounges.
8. A centralized wellness resource center where informational materials on all dimensions of wellness are available on a walk-in basis to students.
9. An accredited wellness major.
10. An increase in the utilization of campus TV, student tapes, and journal articles for the promotion of wellness.
11. An expansion of health-related courses within the health and physical education department.
12. A wellness recess. This is an officially designated time once each semester where people throughout the university are given designated time to investigate one of the dimensions of wellness.
13. Weekly radio spots to promote health-seeking behaviors.
14. Faculty support to encourage responsible use of alcohol.
15. Incentives to increase the activity levels of the students and faculty on campus.
16. More wellness workshops for students and faculty.
17. More opportunities for art to be displayed throughout the campus.
18. More fitness facilities.
19. Whole bran on the tables.
20. Vegetarian entrees that are hot in the grid, such as veggie pastries.
21. Alter the 4-credit physical education requirement with more emphasis on health-related courses.
22. Faculty improvement programs to increase the faculty's participation in personal wellness activities.
23. Improve resident assistant training in dormitories with particular emphasis on encouraging responsible use of alcohol.
24. Encourage the development of alternatives to the square.
25. Develop a wellness-oriented nightclub.
26. Employ student leaders for wellness promotion.
27. Broader bus service and car pooling for students.
28. Dorm representatives for SHAC to insure broad-based support.

29. Assertive training in dorms to improve the environment concerning loud, abusive activities and alcohol-related confusion.
30. Support and encouragement for competitive mental sports.

If there were no student program, UW-SP would still be near the top of the innovators list on the strength of the annual wellness-promotion-strategies conference held each summer in July for the past six years. No other single event, in my opinion, has galvanized, reinforced, and given technical support to the growing number of wellness promoters throughout the U.S. and Canada as has this remarkable "Woodstock of Wellness." The combination of 500 to 600 health-promotion participant enthusiasts, 70-plus faculty members giving presentations and workshops over the course of an entire week, the extremely supportive campus setting in a state acknowledged to be a wellness Mecca, the superb variety of recreational opportunities and the delicious and nutritious foods, all combine to make the experience both unforgettable and addictive. The "Wellness Festival," as it is sometimes called, deserves the praise it receives from everyone who has ever attended as participant or presenter. Except that the latter get their pictures in the program (now distributed to 80,000 people) and give a talk on their special interests in applying wellness, participant and presenter become one in that everyone interacts, presents, listens, and takes from and gives to the festival in his or her unique ways. Which is, of course, in the last analysis, what makes the program so special in the first analysis! If you are free in the third week in July and want to get super-motivated, highly informed, and better connected about all that wellness entails, come to Stevens Point.

All this should not be written without recognizing that a number of administrators, faculty members, students, and outsiders have played key roles in making UW-SP what it is in the wellness movement today. To note a manageable number of such individuals would be almost impossible, though Fred Leafgren and Dennis Elsenrath surely deserve it. However, one special acknowledgment must be given in appreciation of superb contributions to wellness at the UW-SP as well as on a national basis. That, of course, is a kudo to Dr. Bill Hettler, the Director of the Student Health Service from which all of the above is managed. Next to yours truly, Bill is without a doubt the dearest, most lovable, virtuous, and handsome fellow out there proselytizing for wellness.

To get on the mailing list for the annual wellness-strategies-workshop brochure or related information, contact:

Bill Hettler, M.D., Director
Student Health Service
Univ. of Wisc., Delzell Hall
Stevens Point, Wisconsin 54481
(715) 346-4646

WESTERN FEDERAL SAVINGS AND LOAN

Western Federal Savings of Denver is not the oldest, largest, or richest financial institution. But it was the first to develop and carry out a wellness program.

Wellness at Western can be traced to a Gates Foundation conference in late 1978 for business and government leaders in Colorado. The meeting was held at a place called Keystone in the Rocky Mountains; the subject was wellness. In attendance was the president of the association, who was sold on the merits of such a health-promotion enterprise for employees and their families.

At the present time, two years into the program, management is more convinced than ever that wellness has positive consequences for employee morale, work capacity, and a lessening need for medical services. Beyond that, wellness is perceived by management as complementary to good citizenship and a full life. An employee committed to his or her best potentials is, in Western's view, more likely to shape the work environment in order that it be a quality experience. This has obvious consequences for an institution concerned about the quality of interactions between staff and customers.

Responsibility for Western's wellness program is widely shared, but the burden for program design and implementation rests with a wellness committee and a full-time coordinator. In addition to two central Denver locations, Western has twenty-four branches and subsidiaries. A volunteer wellness leader coordinates the program at each of these locations, in addition to his/her regular duties of a banking nature.

At present, the program consists of an assortment of classes, newsletters, juice give-aways, visiting notables, T-shirts, fun runs, and the like. A slide-tape production will soon be available to describe the Western wellness story.

While all this is impressive enough, a new direction is under consideration. A proposal calls for a shift from the current system of targeting limited resources equally throughout the Western system on an omnibus basis of varied offerings. The new approach would call for a centralized system concentrated on a core body of wellness training and leading to some form of certification, recognition, and benefit status. Using this method of standard wellness training, termed a "wellness 101 class series" by the coordinator, all participating Western employees would be encouraged to work toward mastery in all the fundamentals of the five wellness dimensions and the creation of personal wellness plans. Eventually, these might be assessed by a wellness committee and, if consistent with to-be-established Western wellness criteria, be supported by the company via partial subsidies. The latter could take many forms, from membership payments to flex-time arrangements to something else helpful to the employee that does not inhibit timely job performance.

For details on Western wellness procedures, plans, and progress, contact:

Dianne Blachowski, Coordinator
Western Wellness
Western Federal Savings
200 University Boulevard
P.O. Box 5807 T.A.
Denver, Colorado 80217
(303) 370-1212

AID ASSOCIATION FOR LUTHERANS
(Family Health)

Family Health is a health-promotion program of the fraternal benefit society known as Aid Association for Lutherans. Health has been a priority for the insurance-related organization for the nearly 80 years of its existence; since 1977, however, the emphasis has developed to promote wellness in addition to protecting against illness through insurance products. The wellness emphasis is advanced as a member service to millions of individuals through a two-part approach: strengthening family relationships and enhancing personal health. These interlocking agendas are nicely complemented by a variety of products and activities facilitated by a headquarters staff in Appleton, Wisconsin, and implemented through over 5,000 local branches throughout the U.S.

AAL views health as a harmony of the whole, a balance of unique and interdependent relationships between physical, mental, social, and spiritual aspects of the individual in family life. Thus, the entirety of the Family Health wellness endeavor revolves around familial relationships and enhanced personal effectiveness. In the family-relationship arena, six skill areas are emphasized: appreciation for each other, time together, good communication patterns, commitment to each other, high spiritual and religious orientations, and positive ways to deal with crises and problems. In the personal-health focus the dimensions are physical fitness, nutrition, stress management, substance use, safety and medical self-care, and relationships.

The wellness efforts entail the promotion of three kinds of products. The first are awareness products designed to provide knowledge about the wellness option and its myriad attractions. In promotions to date, AAL has gained a national reputation for innovation with the gamelike Wellness Kit. This colorful item has gone over the 50,000 mark in popularity. Also produced as awareness items are wellness booklets and a film.

The second products promoted in the family-health area are informational forums for use at branch meetings. These programs run from 50 to 90 minutes, and include take-home, practical components. The third kinds of products are designed for behavioral-change purposes. These are more complex, and are delivered by para-professional leaders trained by the AAL staff. These are given in the branch setting and run from 10 to 20 hours in length. Other activities include health or wellness fairs and a variety of additional publications on an as-needed basis.

Current directions in Family Health include the development of a family-oriented wellness information system, additional forums on wellness in the context of a fraternal society, design of research and modeling projects for advancing personal and family wellness, and necessary policy supports for establishing wellness as an integral element in the association's family-life-cycle concept.

The implications for variations of the Family Health wellness program by other fraternal and religious organizations are exciting, to put it mildly. If influential groups like this begin to shape their special cultures to reinforce wellness as a natural adjunct to their basic purposes, we could end up with an epidemic of good health.

Wouldn't that be terrific?

For more information about AAL's family-health area write:

Jeffrey R. Hahn
Health Promotion Specialist, Family Health
Aid Association for Lutherans
Appleton, Wisconsin 54919
(414) 734-5721

THE URBAN COUNCIL ON ADOLESCENCE AND WELLNESS (UCAW)

One of the most predictable questions when taking inquiries following a talk on the wellness concept is, "What is being done to make these concepts available to disadvantaged populations?" For the most part, wellness is a lifestyle embraced by and available to middle- and upper-class folks with good educations and generally favorable environmental circumstances. Until 1979, when the Urban Council got underway, there was little of substance to talk about concerning wellness in areas still struggling with the lower items on Maslow's hierarchy. The Urban Council merits a lot of talking (or writing) about.

The basic purpose of the Council is to promote an awareness of, and a commitment to, the wellness lifestyle for the young people in the Greater Newark, New Jersey, area. It is less a direct service effort than a center and facilitator for a vast range of service organizations. These include business corporations, foundations, public agencies, schools, and churches. The focus is on individual and cultural change; a guiding intent is to establish wellness as the norm for the majority rather than a difficult-to-sustain breakthrough success story for a few high achievers.

The philosophy of the Urban Council is set forth in its charter. It is dedicated to holistic approaches to total (psychological as well as physical) health, and to the training and maximum use of peer wellness counselors. It also seeks cooperation with local and state agencies in dealing with teenage health problems, in designing and carrying out a continuing series of needed educational forums, and in raising the health status of adolescents. In summary, UCAW attempts to serve as a public advocate for area young and to promote and advance the idea of high-level wellness in every way possible.

Council materials reveal a strong belief in the uniqueness of each adolescent, and in the special opportunities which this period of life affords for making wise choices that can guide and shape a life direction of meaning and purpose. The overriding emphasis is clearly on the aspect of self-responsibility, and all that entails.

The Council operates a multidisciplinary wellness resource center, publishes a resource directory and a teen newsletter, and conducts individual programs in each of the five wellness dimensions, plus a sixth which cultivates the capacity for relating to and communicating with others. It coordinates with the Frost Valley YMCA to send hundreds of inner-city youth to the Catskills each summer for weeks of outdoor adventures, advanced wellness training and environmental sensitivity. Problem situations are dealt with in a variety of interesting ways (such as role playing). A lot of attention is given to learning to deal with peers in satisfying but nonadversarial ways. Hundreds of youngsters have gone through the DISCO (Discussing Intelligently Self and other Concerns Openly) program. Skits and dialogues on the range of issues that come out of these interactions have been performed for many audiences in the area. Many workshops on special problem areas (such as teen pregnancy) have been sponsored for other agencies and groups. Models for teen self-development have been created, "feeling good" fitness programs have been started through the Council in different grade schools; and many young people in the area have been exposed to the running themes of the wellness program that consist of "self-responsibility, self-respect, and self-esteem." It has even reached the point where local judges in some instances remand youngsters to the DISCO program, with reasonably encouraging results to date.

A great deal of the momentum, innovation, and public acceptance is due to Robert L. Johnson, M.D., Director of Adolescent Medicine at the New Jersey Medical School; Howard Quirk, head of the Victoria Foundation; and Elizabeth Allston, Executive Director of the Urban Council since its inception in 1979. There is much to be done — in many ways it is still getting off the ground, but the Council already enjoys recognition and acceptance both within and beyond the community it serves.

For service to and advancement of the wellness ethic within the less-advantaged community, there is nothing quite like the Urban Council to date.

For details, contact:

Ms. Liz Allston, Program Manager
Urban Council on Adolescence and Wellness
Protest Community Center Inc.
19 James Street
Newark, New Jersey, 07102
(201) 483-0317

REALISTIC HYGIENE

"A wellness lifestyle has oral implications." That is the view of John Duffy, founder and head of an organization that has conducted dental-wellness workshops for years throughout the Midwest and who has described in practical terms the nature of such implications for thousands of people since starting his program.

Dental-wellness workshops are short courses in oral health promotion. People learn not only how to recognize mouth problems in early stages and what causes tooth and gum disease, but also develop the skills needed to minimize problems by maximizing their prospects for enjoyable oral well-being. As with healthy lifestyle practices in each of the five dimensions (which are reinforced at all of the workshops), Dr. Duffy believes the best payoffs which sustain superb oral practices and habits over a lifetime are omnipresent, near-term rewards (e.g., great smiles, positive image, and a mouth that feels alive and fresh).

The wellness workshops conducted for companies and other large groups of people utilize lectures, small group experiential sessions, and individual practices which are supervised and professionally evaluated.

The program is particularly valuable to companies who have, or are contemplating, dental insurance, the employee benefit that helps people live *with* their dental problems. The Dental Wellness

Workshop can help them live *without* dental problems, a real benefit to employees, and a cost savings to employers.

Realistic Hygiene particularly enjoys doing this program for teachers as a way of multiplying their efforts. If enough teachers understood and practiced the principles of dental wellness, then oral-health-education programs for students could become truly effective and help the next generation avoid the world's most prevalent health problem — dental disease.

Realistic Hygiene may be one way to look at the future for a good part of dental education. It represents a unique approach to *oral* health promotion by translating the very kind of positive approaches that are working so well to motivate other lifestyle-based wellness programs. It is cost-effective, gives predictable results, fits nicely with other individual or group medical and wellness programs, and is highly desired and appreciated by the people who experience the training.

To learn more, write John Duffy at:

Realistic Hygiene, Inc.
2354 Highway AB
McFarland, Wisconsin 53558
(608) 838-8700

GREATER MILWAUKEE CONFERENCE ON RELIGION AND URBAN AFFAIRS

The GMCRUA is an interfaith organization that serves as a vehicle for the participation of the organized religious community in urban issues throughout the Greater Milwaukee area. Since 1977, the Conference has supported a task force whose mission has been to help churches and synagogues promote individual and community wellness. The Wholistic Health Care Task Force is comprised of about 25 professionals from social service, business, clergy and medical backgrounds. These people devote time because they feel a personal commitment to wellness and a conviction that congregations have a unique opportunity and ability to promote wellness through shared spiritual values.

The task force, and the larger GMCRUA, believes that wellness is rooted in Judeo-Christian theology. Churches and synagogues traditionally have advocated wholeness of body, mind and spirit, and have ministered to the needs of individuals seeking these processes that hold central the need for purpose and meaning in life. Religion can be a source of inspiration and provide a community of support for the pursuit and attainment of wholeness and well-being.

In advancing these purposes, the task force has enabled the GMCRUA to establish and support "congregational teams" at local levels, to assess needs, conduct classes, sponsor regional seminars, and work as a catalyst and guide in providing resources for individual churches and synagogues. Their most recent project is a Wellness Volunteer Training Program which introduces congregational members to wellness theory, group-process skills and program planning so that wellness programs can be more expansive and ongoing.

This is an extraordinary development, not because of the achievements of the task force and the GMCRUA (which have certainly been notable), but because of the precedent established. If this pattern of religious support and advocacy for wellness spreads in the future (and inquiries to the GMCRUA suggest that this is already happening), then yet another massive wave of assistance for awareness of health enhancement as an integral part of the whole life will be realized.

For more information about the task force and GMCRUA:

Karen Schudson, Coordinator
Wholistic Health Care Task Force
Greater Milwaukee Conference on Religion & Urban Affairs
1442 N. Farwell Avenue
Milwaukee, Wisconsin 53202

ALLEN MEMORIAL HOSPITAL
Waterloo, Iowa

Waterloo, Iowa? How does it happen that some of the most advanced wellness initiatives are taken in places few have heard of? One reason might be that there are fewer bureaucratic obstacles to overcome; another may be the presence of underestimated levels of progressive-minded leaders in small off-the-worn path locations in the "Heartland". One certain explanation for the presence and quality of the Wellness Center at Allen Memorial Hospital is James A. Schlueter, the program director and nationally known wellness promoter hired to establish a wellness outpost in Waterloo.

After only one year, Allen Memorial Hospital has a Wellness Center operating in the black, that is making more money than it spends or costs! This is unprecedented — and when word gets out look for a stream of wellness center delegations heading for Iowa. (The local dirt airstrip may soon be renamed Waterloo International.) For information, write:

James A. Schlueter, Director
Wellness Center
Allen Memorial Hospital
1825 Logan Ave.
Waterloo, IA 50703
319-235-3615

SENTRY INSURANCE

Sentry Insurance in Stevens Point, Wisconsin, is the Mercedes-Benz of the corporate wellness world. In addition to enjoying proximity to the University of Wisconsin-Stevens Point Wellness Activity Center and a spectacular building and site in a wooded environment, Sentry has a superb program staffed with highly trained, experienced leaders in the health-promotion field. Sentry employees also have available, as part of this "too-good-to-miss" package, a multi-million-dollar fitness center with everything imaginable — and more. (A list of all this would take too much space!)

Sentry's program is based on a five-part philosophy:

1. Mentally, emotionally and physically fit employees are of more value to themselves, their families, and their employer.
2. Such employees have less absenteeism, become more productive and generally require less illness care or disability expenditures.
3. Healthy lifestyles and practices increase quality as well as quantity of life and should be largely self-directed.
4. The working environment should be both safe and conducive to health improvement.
5. Employees have a right to choose which, if any, health activities in which they wish to participate.

The stated objectives which lead to the realization of these goals reveals the comprehensive nature of the program:

1. Adequate physical activity and rest with an emphasis on aerobic activities to increase the efficiency with which oxygen is delivered to the brain, heart and other parts of the body.
2. Proper nutrition including the U.S. Dietary Goals of weight control, dietary balance, decreased intake of saturated fats, cholesterol, salt, simple carbohydrates and red meat, and increased use of complex carbohydrates (fiber), fish, poultry and legumes.
3. Control of smoking, alcohol, caffeine, and medication or drug usage. Smoking cessation group programs are offered regularly and alcohol moderation is stressed especially at holiday seasons.
4. Understanding of stress and its management including improvement of family and business interpersonal relations.
5. Proper use of health professionals such as doctors and nurses with information on appropriateness of self-care.
6. Personalized "adaptive" programs for those with special circumstances.

Eligibility is extended to all employees working at least half-time, their spouses and dependents, retirees, and guests of employees. Virtually, 100% of the eligible work force at World Headquarters is exposed to company media regarding health promotion. Over 90% choose the prevention-oriented HMO plan for illness and injury care, and increasing numbers of people with disabilities take part in the "adaptive" program.

Sentry's wellness effort features a wide range of program choices, a monthly publication, extensive assessments, the availability of counseling on varied issues, flexible work hours, participation credits, a medical self-care module, and a rigorous evaluation component.

Don Johnson, M.D., the director of the program, feels that the key to long-lasting behavior change is a strong belief in the wisdom of that change, coupled with an ongoing supportive environment. To that end, employees are encouraged to adopt healthier lifestyles only when the idea makes sense to them. Thus, a low-key approach marks the Sentry endeavor.

For more information on the aspects noted above, write:

Don Johnson
Vice President and Medical Director
Sentry Insurance
1800 North Point Drive
Stevens Point, Wisconsin 54481
(715) 346-7450

CONTINENTAL HEALTH EVALUATION CENTER

Wellness is the watchword at the 388-acre residential complex about 25 miles north of Denver and 10 miles east of Boulder. CHEC is staffed by a team of physicians, exercise physiologists, physical therapists, nutritionists, psychologists and others committed to integrating wellness lifestyle teachings with medical management of an array of degenerative conditions — e.g., coronary-artery disease, hypertension, arthritis, adult onset of diabetes, peripheral vascular disease, obesity, etc. CHEC is part vacation resort, part boot camp, and part university. It is wholly devoted to independent, client-centered shaping of lifestyle patterns for optimal functioning after the individual leaves the program.

The facilities are superb; the food is both nutritious and delicious; and the program is vigorous and varied. However, three features of the CHEC 26-Day Residential Program (at about $4,200) distinguish it from the better-known model which inspired the Colorado edition (the Longevity Institute in Santa Monica): (1) staff enthusiasm for wellness; (2) a focus on the development of inner-directed behavior change; and (3) a spectacular location at the foot of the Rocky Mountains.

The program attends to all five wellness dimensions, with a focus on nutritional awareness, physical fitness, and stress management. The diet is 80-85% complex carbohydrates, 15-18% protein, and only about 6% fat. In this regard, CHEC out-Pritikins Pritikin! The following menu is typical of the meal pattern and educational style at CHEC.*

---

*As the second edition of this book went to press, we learned that the Continental Health Evaluation Center has since gone out of business.

SAMPLE OF ACTUAL MENU

BREAKFAST	AMT.	CAL.	FAT	PROT.	CARB.	NA.	CHOL.
Grapefruit	½	40	—	—	10	1	—
Spanish Omelette	3 egg whites	110	3	14	5	216	20
Toast	1 slice	50	—	2	11	1	—
Apple Butter	1 T.	20	—	—	5	2	—
TOTALS		220	3gm	16gm	31gm	220mg	20mg

Which breakfast will you eat when you get home?

BREAKFAST	AMT.	CAL.	FAT	PROT.	CARB.	NA.	CHOL.
Bacon	3 Sl.	147	13	5	—	250	21
Fried Eggs	2	216	17	12	1	338	520
Toast	1 Sl.	140	—	4	30	200	—
Butter	1 T.	108	12	—	—	124	30
TOTALS		611	42gm	21gm	31gm	912mg*	571mg

Dinner (supper) is the lightest meal of the day; breakfast and lunch are substantial. All three are delicious (which I state from personal experience). Here is a sample dinner menu with educational tidbits included.

SUPPER	AMT.	CAL.	FAT	PROT.	CARB.	NA.	CHOL.
Pita Bread Sandwich	2 Halves	200	—	4	34	(4)	—
Sunshine	½ c.	52	.2	2.5	10.9	23	—
TOTALS		252	.2gm	6.5gm	44.9gm	27mg	

Delicious food somehow seems all the more enjoyable when you are free of concerns about the after effects of what you are eating.

---

*Those restricting sodium should be aware that the sodium content of some fast foods is extremely high. A medium-size pizza from Pizza Hut, for instance, may contain more than 4,000 mg. of sodium. A Dairy Queen Brazier Dog with cheese may contain 1986 mg. of sodium, while a McDonald's Big Mac may contain 962 mg. of sodium. (Source: Sue Hicks, CHEC Nutritionist.)

A lot of attention is given to outcome evaluation, that is, assessments of the extent to which the 26-Day experience made a substantive difference in the health of clients. Thus, all participants are given thorough assessments during and after the visit. The usual wellness vital signs are assessed (e.g., pulse rate, body composition, oxygen-utilization capacity) in addition to important medical checks (e.g., cholesterol, HDL, and other blood measures).

The best insights about CHEC come from conversations with the staff. For example, I loved the explanation offered by Tashof Bernton, M.D., as to why so much attention is given to challenging games, activities, and other almost playful group endeavors: "Being sick is serious business; if you can't be serious, it is hard to stay sick." "Tash" also mentioned that the source of his satisfaction at CHEC is the continuing opportunity to work with a cross section of clients. (Unlike yours truly — when I give lectures, the audience is usually 99% super-healthy types. The joggers, vegetarians, meditators, and others already well along the wellness path all show up to hear what a great thing it is that they are making such good lifestyle choices. Thus, my audiences consist of the true believers — the choir of wellness.) "It is more challenging to work with older, sicker, overweight folks than the no-nukes, save-the-whales, vegetarian healthies," notes "Tash."

Robert Swearingen, M.D., consultant, believes that the challenge at CHEC (and elsewhere) is to stimulate in clients some internally produced vitamin, mineral, chemical or other mysterious element which he terms "substance X." Studies of joggers and other groups characterized by commitment to health-enhancing practices suggest that some kind of chemical reactions occur in these instances which fill the adherents with enthusiasm and high levels of self-esteem. This has been called a placebo in the past; whether imaginary or real, the mood and results at CHEC suggest something happens (substance X or just effective preparation) to help guests to enhance their health and enthusiasm generated during their residence at Continental Health.

Everyone receives a wellness report at the conclusion of the program. Though impressed with the range and intensity of the activities, the diet, the enthusiasm of the staff, and other characteristics of CHEC, the summary report may be the best feature of the entire endeavor. It is designed to help the participant "put it all together," and the chances are good that it does just that. It relates the key data to lifestyle-change suggestions based on the during the residential period. The summary is a series of personal letters from each of the experts responsible for one or more of the five wellness dimensions. Finally, the manual also serves as a final pep talk, expressed in a caring manner that grows out of the close relationships that evolve between clients and facilitators. If all this does not work, my guess is that the unaffected character is, at least for wellness purposes, a lost cause. Fortunately, it seems that follow-up checks indicate there have been few such write-offs in the first year of CHEC's existence as a first-class wellness retreat and learning center.

It was a surprise to learn that CHEC is sometimes referred to as "Colorado's best-kept secret." Something should be done to rectify this. If you have an interest in a unique wellness-oriented vacation, recovery period, or training, you might "check" this one out. For information, write or call:

Continental Health Evaluation Center
4801 N. 107th Street
Lafayette, Colorado 80026
(303) 665-9020

INTERFACE

Interface is a not-for-profit organization in Newton, Ma. devoted to the promotion of wellness lifestyles. In operation since 1974, the agency has evolved from a holistic medicine oriented center to a broader based educational forum. The goal at Interface is to help people assume responsibility for their own well being — physically, emotionally, mentally, and spiritually — and to recognize their innate capacity for self healing and personal growth. Offerings range from brief evening lectures to in-depth training sessions over a period of weeks. Last year, more than 230 programs were offered; the budget for the coming year anticipates participation by at least 10,000 in Interface programs. A Master's degree program is provided in cooperation with Beacon College in Holistic Education. An annual meeting on holistic health is held in November which attracts hundreds of practitioners and lay people from throughout North America.

For information about Interface, write or call:

Rose Thorn, Executive Director
Interface
230 Central Street
Newton, Ma 02166
(617) 964-7140

A WELLNESS COMMUNITY/RETREAT

Rumors have it that John Travis, M.D., founder of the world's first wellness resource center, has dropped out. It has even been said that he moved to a jungle in South America! And, furthermore, that he has established an "intentional community" focused on alternative energy and self sufficiency, spiritual growth, material simplicity, and the interconnectedness between all life forms. The rumors are true, with one exception: he has not dropped out — he just stepped aside, temporarily, to reflect and explore in order to grow in directions that seem important to him. These include a complex of issues related to wellness that probably will be "hot" in the year 2000 — and maybe a lot sooner. The site of the good doctor's living laboratory is Costa Rica in Central America, in a small settlement called Ojala, about 100 miles from the capitol of San Jose.

Far from dropping out, Dr. Travis travels a lecture circuit three months out of the year, produces a newsletter on a regular basis to subscribers, and conducts retreats throughout the year at Ojala on all the issues noted above related to "planetary wellness." Furthermore, his workbooks (see review of the Wellness Workbook in Part Three) are continuing to help shape the thinking of thousands of people throughout the country and thus to influence more than a few wellness programs.

For information about Travis' newsletter, workbooks, lectures and/or the community/retreat at Ojala, write or call:
Wellness Associates
Suite A
42 Miller Avenue
Mill Valley, Ca 94941
(415) 383-3806

MADISON MEMORIAL HIGH SCHOOL

The second most often asked question posed at the wellness seminars which I conduct in various and sundry places (after the question about what is being done to make wellness information more accessible to and feasible for disadvantaged populations) is: "Why is wellness not taught in the schools?" The answer is that it should be and soon will be widely available at all levels — and has been for years a required course at one high school in Madison, Wisconsin.

Wellness began at Memorial because of the leadership of then-principal, Dr. Richard Schafer. What began as fun runs, optional after-school discussion groups and activities, and additions to standardized health education and physical fitness classes, soon branched out into other disciplines and school activities as more teachers and students were attracted to the varied programs organized by Dr. Schafer. These included a few day-long wellness workshops for both students and teachers from throughout the area. Soon, the students began requesting more on these kinds of health enhancement options, a parcourse was constructed, and the scene was set for wellness to be integrated into the curricula.

At present, all students must pass a course on the fundamentals of the wellness concept prior to graduation. More important, the range of opportunities for participation has been greatly expanded, the level of involvement is high, and the students themselves are the ones who are shaping the educational culture at Madison Memorial. Today, it is more likely than ever before that others coming along will find health-enhancing alternatives to be both attractive and plentiful.

The Madison program does not provide all the answers; no one at the school would suggest otherwise. However, it does, unintentionally, raise a number of questions in my mind and probably yours, too. Why is wellness not a required subject in all schools? Why *not* encourage youngsters to start a personal wellness-plan process when important habit patterns are being formed, some of which will last a lifetime? Why *not* have as a goal for all schools the promotion of wellness lifestyles that could assist each youngster to feel liked, valued, able, and worthy? Why not do everything possible to eliminate or at least moderate guilt and worry to the extent possible? Why not pull out all stops to build self-confidence and to undermine self-defeating behaviors? Schools should, in this view, be concerned about helping young people function effectively in an imperfect world. Schools should be as committed to providing opportunities for wellness as they are to transmitting knowledge in other areas. The Madison experience may, in a later analysis, be valued more for what it encouraged others to do than for what it achieved, however commendable this role has been.

Tips for starting school wellness programs and related assistance is available by writing or calling:

Richard O. Schafer, Ph.D., Executive Director
Lifestyle 80s
P.O. Box 5069
Madison, Wisconsin 53705
(608) 833-4476

WELLNESS INSTITUTES

Throughout the U.S. and Canada, a number of training programs are developing which offer residential wellness experiences. For a set fee, such institutes provide information about getting started with health-enhancing lifestyles. Most last for five or more days (though all offer variations and related products) and use faculty on contract.

SUN VALLEY HEALTH INSTITUTE

Founded in 1973 in Sun Valley, Idaho, in a small hospital oriented to the casualties of the famous ski runs, SVHI was, until very recently, an executive testing and health hazard avoidance program in the classic prevention mold. Approximately 3,000 persons, mostly business executives (and spouses) participated in the once- or twice-annual residence programs during the early years.

With the recent advance of the wellness movement, however, the Institute has begun to expand and extend its efforts, giving special focus to the provision of assistance to hospital-based, health-promotion endeavors. SVHI now offers, for example, a package of consultation, education, and training options to hospitals getting involved in such efforts. By 1985, the Institute expects to be working on a contract basis with 150 community hospitals in 20 states.

The SVHI program includes video modules on a variety of prevention and health promotion topics, as well as a risk factor assessment profile, and a facilitator's guide or instructor's manual for conducting the Institute's program. In addition, the Institute has compiled a *Health Guide* for participants. Program evaluations, in terms of individual outcomes after the trainings, are conducted at 30-90 day intervals; a quarterly newsletter is sent to all participants; and marketing advice is available for those hospitals which sign up for the programs.

For cost or other information about this model, write or call:

Gary R. Steinbach, President
Sun Valley Health Institute
P.O. Box 1720
Sun Valley, Idaho 83353
(208) 622-5343

WALLINGFORD WELLNESS PROJECT

Wellness applies to everybody, but carrying out the principles and techniques of this philosophy invites adaptations for special groups. This section has described a number of creative wellness programs for such diverse groups as the very young, minorities, poor, religious interests, women, and so on. But, what about the elderly? Is there an existing model for focusing wellness within the unique context of the aged?

There is. In Seattle, Washington.

The Wallingford Wellness Project is a wellness program for older people. It is led by participants who graduated from the earliest classes. The key lesson of Wallingford is that older people bring to a wellness program a lifetime of experience, skills, time, energy, and enthusiasm as program leaders fully capable of cultivating the seeds of wellness for others in the community.

The program focuses on the five wellness dimensions. Everyone involved is both a learner and a leader. Graduates teach new participants, who in turn work with their peers and neighbors on ways to develop and live a wellness lifestyle.

The program managers have further extended the Wallingford experience by providing workshops for trainers and program developers across North America. A variety of resource materials, including a slide tape show about Wallingford, is available to groups interested in starting their own community-based wellness programs for elderly people.

For information, contact:

Stephanie J. FallCreek
Wallingford Wellness Project
School of Social Work, M.S. JH-30
University of Washington
4101 15th Ave. N.E.
Seattle, Wa. 98195
(206) 545-1632

PLANNING FOR WELLNESS, INC.

Planning for Wellness is an Oregon corporation organized to present seminars, train wellness educators, and produce books and videotapes on all the wellness dimensions.

The company has produced the following materials in the past year:

"A Personal Plan for Wellness" — a thirty minute video co-sponsored by U.S. National Bank of Oregon. The show describes the key steps involved in personal wellness planning and follows a family as they struggle to improve their health habits. The tape includes a comprehensive instructor's guide.

"Wellness Lifestyles" — a thirty minute video/film in conjunction with ABC Video Enterprises. The film introduces the wellness concept and covers self-responsibility, nutrition, fitness, stress management, and environmental sensitivity. Features former astronaut Edgar Mitchell, Bess Meyerson, Drs. Tager and Ardell.

Planning for Wellness: A Guidebook for Optimal Health published by Kendall/Hunt Publishers (second edition). This popular workbook assists the reader in developing a personal wellness plan to be used at home, work and play. The guidebook is currently being used by many corporations, schools and hospitals in North America.

The company is presently developing additional videotapes and films for cable and public broadcast.

For Information Write or Call:
Planning for Wellness
2731 SW 2nd
Portland, Oregon 97201
(503) 295-5952 or
(415) 383-0976

THUNDER BAY DISTRICT HEALTH COUNCIL

From 1976-1978, when the leading institutional promoters of wellness lifestyles were health-planning agencies, the Canadian counterparts of U.S. health-system agencies (HSAs) were the Ontario district health councils. Though smaller in terms of staff and other resources, the interest level for many of the DHCs was comparable to the innovations being realized by American planners. In 1979, when the latter agencies were directed by federal officials to concentrate on regulatory matters and cost-control issues and drop the health promotion endeavors, the Canadian DHCs found themselves in a lead role in pioneering wellness strategies from the unique perspective and role of the health-planning agency.

Far and away the most active of the DHCs in promoting wellness from day one has been the Thunder Bay DHC, led by C. Wesley Leicester, the executive director of the agency. Because of his commitment and the support of similarly enthusiastic board members, the TBDHC has been able to compile a record of initiative that would make proud even the most ardent wellness planner.

Among the achievements to date have been a vast range of public awareness programs on wellness, such as seminars, workshops tailored to special groups (e.g., homemakers, employers), entire plan sections on ways to implement wellness into public policy, and a variety of fitness campaigns involving large numbers of people in different cities.

Today, when the U.S. HSAs have become irrelevant, no longer supported by the current administration because they are judged ineffective at cost control and uninvolved in health promotion (though, ironically, the previous administration forced them out of this area), DHCs are prospering with a wellness orientation. Nowhere is there a better planning model as to what can be and what is being done than in the far northern reaches of Thunder Bay, Ontario.

For more on the DHC role in wellness, contact:

C. Wesley Leicester, Executive Director
Thunder Bay District Health Council
Suite 1, 516 Victoria Avenue
Thunder Bay F,
Ontario P7C 1A7
Canada

THE STAY WELL PLAN*

Blue Shield of California developed an experimental self-care and wellness-incentive program on the premise that most people have abdicated personal responsibility for their own health. This abdication is the result of a growing conviction on the part of the individual that he cannot do much to help himself, and a lack of real concern as to the cost of the medical care he believes he needs. The result has been a continued increase in utilization of health-care facilities and personnel. This has led to a rapid growth of facilities and trained personnel to meet the increased demand. This growth-demand cycle has made health-care costs a major economic problem.

Blue Shield believes there are three major components in the cost of health care: inflation, utilization and technology. Controlling or slowing the rising cost of health care means controlling at least one of these factors. Inflation is a worldwide phenomenon and beyond the scope of individual effort. The advance of medical technology is considered essential, and slowing its development might be counter-productive. Utilization of medical care, however, is a different matter since it is essentially an individual determination. While the individual cannot control cost, he can

---

*Parts of this account are edited excerpts from Blue Shield Materials.

and does control the decision to buy. It is here we believe we can exercise effective cost containment.

The "Stay Well Plan" is about the control of utilization.

The Patient and the Doctor

Medical economists estimate that as much as 50%-70% of physician-patient contacts are unnecessary. Most visits to a doctor or hospital emergency room are for treatment of self-limiting conditions, such as the common cold, flu, upset stomach and the like. This use of medical care places a severe strain on both financial and medical resources.

It is estimated that the average family of four will see a physician or use a hospital emergency room approximately 12 times a year. If only half of these visits are unnecessary, these families are wasting not only a substantial amount of their own financial resources and time, but are utilizing medical resources needed for the more seriously ill. Moreover, to the extent that production or job time is lost while the employee seeks medical care, additional cost must be added to the health-care package.

It has been determined that the decision to seek medical care is based, first, on how the individual views his medical problem; second, on the availability of care; and, lastly, on the cost of that care. If the problem is perceived as serious, if medical care is readily available and if health insurance or other resources are sufficient to meet all or most of the cost, the decision to seek medical care is almost automatic. In fact, the existence of any two of these conditions will likely result in a decision to seek care. Conversely, the lack of any two of these factors will likely result in a negative decision.

It is generally agreed that reasonable availability of medical care is a desirable condition. Therefore, control of unnecessary utilization will depend on our ability to influence how the individual views his need for care (and ultimately the cause of his ill health), and the resources necessary to pay for care.

The "Stay Well Plan" provides the individual with understandable and practical information that will assist him in determining need for care and a strong positive incentive to properly utilize this information.

The program is divided into two steps. First, the employee is given health-promotion information to assist him to take care of himself and make proper use of medical care, and second, he is offered a cash incentive for staying well. For step one, the employee gets a copy of *Take Care of Youself, a Consumer's Guide to Medical Care,* along with information on how to utilize the book. This book provides a practical guide to identification of most common medical problems. It illustrates the nature of problems, when and how to use home care, and when to see a doctor. It is supplemented by a monthly newsletter containing further information on self-care.

The uniqueness and genuine innovation of the "stay well" program is with step two. A sum of $500 (it can be any set amount) is deposited for each employee to pay the first $500 of covered medical expense that he and/or his family require. (The employee's group-health coverage pays for expenses in excess of $500.) If the employee or his family remain well (i.e., do not utilize all or a portion of the first $500) for the next 12 months, these monies are returned to him in cash. This approach not only reinforces the idea of personal responsibility for his own health, but in effect lets the employee insure himself for the first $500 of covered medical expense. It provides an incentive for shaping a wellness lifestyle!

In these two steps the employee is given both the tools and the incentive to utilize medical care properly and to avoid unnecessary care. An employer may select the educational component alone, or both the educational and incentive components. If this program reduces the number of unnecessary physician-patient contacts by as little as 25%, and if necessary medical care is sought promptly, there will be a dramatic reduction in the cost of medical care to both the employee and the employer.

For the facts about program mechanics, costs, and results to date, contact:

Charles L. Parcell
Vice-President
Blue Shield of California
2 North Point
San Francisco, California 94133
(415) 445-5084

SACRED HEART HOSPITAL

A variation on "Stay Well" is underway in Yankton, South Dakota. At Sacred Heart Hospital, an employee who thinks he is too well to go to work can call in healthy! Really. Naturally, this is quite a shift from the established sickness consciousness that follows the standard benefit packages that offer two or three weeks paid leave for sickness each year and no incentives for health or behaviors likely to keep you that way. At Sacred Heart, a small hospital with only 400 employees, individuals are awarded three "well days" a year for good attendance and health habits. Such days can be taken as time off or cash; savings of either are permitted. Obviously, the system provides a modest but welcome inducement for wellness living. Look for more of this kind of creative benefit for workers in the near future.

For more about the Sacred Heart approach and results, write:

Bill Blount, RPT
Sacred Heart Hospital
Yankton, S.D. 57078
(605) 665-9371

THE LIFEGAIN PROGRAM

When the roll is called up yonder or anywhere else to give awards for promoting wellness, Robert Allen and the Lifegain program will be at or near the head of the line. Lifegain is a carefully arranged systems approach for changing those parts of the culture which people find inhibiting to a wellness lifestyle. It is patterned on an earlier program called Normative Systems, which Dr. Allen's Human Resources Institute developed and administered over a 20-year time span during the course of about 600 engagements. The Lifegain program, addressed to the five wellness dimensions and a few others thrown in for good measure, is the single most popular mechanism for organizing an institutional wellness program. It is, as of the end of 1981, in use at 20 hospital-based wellness centers and an additional 80 locations, such as companies, service organizations, and other public and private entities.

What accounts for the popularity of Lifegain? A lot of things. Let me count a few of the reasons. First, there is the emphasis on changing not just the individual but the larger cultures of which he/she is a part — and which constitute the true variables in whether lifestyle reform can survive the passage of the good intentions phase. Without culture change, long-term resolutions fare poorly. Second, Lifegain offers a complete package of ready-to-use materials from leader manuals to detailed booklets on the basics of wellness in all its dimensions and forms. Thus, it is convenient and easy to implement. Third, it is mainstream in style and content. The material is well researched: Lifegain avoids blame placing, an over-emphasis on initial motivation, the usual appeal to individual heroics, a focus on activities rather than results, reliance on unapplied knowledge, and a "We can do it for you" attitude. A fourth reason for Lifegain's surge to the top of the charts as a hit way to organize wellness is that it has great principles that work, such as a commitment to personal involvement, caring for others, a health rather than an illness emphasis, attention to sound data and measurable results, freedom of choice, and a characteristic of sustained achievement and a fun orientation as the key measures of the system. There are other reasons, no doubt: it is inexpensive, it is well tried, and it allows managers to start a program with confidence but still affords great spaces for individual creativity in shaping individual programs around the broad outine model. But there is one other reason that has to be acknowledged because it surely is as much of a factor in the Lifegain success story as any of the others. That, of course, is the presence of Robert Allen as the head of the Lifegain program and its chief (low-key) salesman, who is a very articulate and persuasive model for the Lifegain system and the wellness lifestyle.

Two of Dr. Allen's books are reviewed and recommended on the Honor Roll of recommended publications found in the back of this work. One of the two books is about Lifegain.

For more about Lifegain, write or call:

Human Resources Institute, (HRI)
Tempe Wick Road
Morristown, New Jersey 07960
(201) 267-1496

Part Three

The Honor Roll of Recommended Books

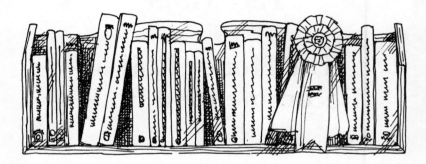

Part Three

The Honor Roll of Recommended Books

There is so much to wellness. One special quality of this kind of approach to health is that you never need worry that there is no more to learn. There is, and always will be.

Each wellness dimension has unbounded possibilities. It would be easy enough to fill an average-sized public library with books devoted exclusively to any of the five dimensions. However, you will always have favorites — books that inspire, clarify, entertain, and otherwise enable you to go farther and enjoy more in one or all of the key wellness areas. I certainly do, and I want to share my list with you. Each of these books helped me at some stage of my journey to new adventures in well-being; maybe many of them will be useful for you.

You may be somewhat interested in the criteria I used to decide if a book deserved inclusion on my Wellness Honor Roll. For starters, it had to be interesting and persuasive, and it was essential that the author demonstrated some appreciation for the importance of lifestyle as a principle determinant of health. In addition, I looked for a non-dogmatic attitude, an awareness of more than a single dimension (though the book might be devoted to nutrition or fitness), and a sense of humor. If the author was a physician, I watched closely for signs of condescension or an unwillingness to give responsibility to the reader. Perhaps most important, I tried to be aware of how I felt during and after reading the book. Was I excited about taking new initiatives, testing new knowledge gained, and exploring new realizations and strategies for my own well-being? If so, the book was destined for the list.

You might consider developing your own honor roll of wellness books, in accord with your own criteria, which may or may not be similar to my selections and evaluation. In any event, I would be interested in hearing from you regarding your assessment of any book which deserves Honor Roll status (write care of the publisher).

Self-Responsibility

Ardell, Donald B. *High Level Wellness: An Alternative to Doctors, Drugs, and Disease.* Emmaus, Pa. and New York: Rodale Press and Bantam Books, 1977 and 1979.

The task of assessing this book was as difficult as the critique of any other review appearing on the honor roll. After all, I know the author — what would people think? Could I be objective?

Well, people will think what they are going to think. In any event, I dealt with the objectivity issue by deciding not to be objective. Since I am interested in how I perceive *High Level Wellness* several years after writing it, I thought you might be also.

High Level Wellness: An Alternative to Doctors, Drugs, and Disease was the first publication on the nature of a wellness lifestyle designed to encourage the reader to pursue his or her highest potentials for well-being. It introduced the five dimensions and ten principles of wellness, contained a description of innovative holistic health and the Wellness Resource Centers, highlighted wellness programs in industry, and listed ways that committed individuals could band together for a healthier society. As with this book, *High Level Wellness* provided an "honor roll" of recommended publications for the reader desirous of more material in each of the five dimensions.

Strengths

I believed at the time that the strength of the book was to be found in the general theme that wellness is a richer way to be alive, that it provides its own reward, and that the pursuit of a health-enhancing lifestyle in individualized ways makes possible a richer integration of your physical, mental and emotional potentials. This perspective has not changed. My favorite part of the book is the ten principles, though I am also well pleased with the substantive discussion and recommendations in each of the five basic wellness dimensions.

Weaknesses

There are many things I would do differently if writing the same book today. I would downplay the attention given to holistic-health centers, be a bit less harsh on doctors, and eliminate a good number of wellness measures (e.g., the voice stress analysis). There would be lots of changes in the nutrition section. Not all the books listed in the honor roll of recommended publications would stay there, and there would be some changes in all the other wellness dimensions in terms of specific recommendations. Part of these changes would be due to a changed perspective in my knowledge about certain issues, others would be related to developments in the past year or so (e.g., the New England Holistic Health Center is no longer in existence), and the majority would simply reflect my own evolution in thinking about and shaping my own wellness lifestyle.

If you read this book, guard against the "swallow-it-whole" syndrome. It is surprising how many people get trapped in an all-or-nothing point of view, which can cost the loss of new ideas here and there. I sometimes encounter someone who says, "I loved your work, until you mentioned Adelle Davis" or "wheat germ" or whatever. Why get hung up on the parts you do not like? Go with what applies and makes sense to you, and forget the rest. Incidentally, I reread the book for this review and was pleased to note that I still believe 80 percent of the material is solid — right on target. Perhaps 15 percent is marginal or dull, and only five percent is out-and-out dangerous nonsense! Not bad — Hoffer once said that a book is worthwhile if you get *one* good idea from it. (No, I cannot tell you *which* five percent I refer to and no, you cannot get a five percent discount.) The wellness dimensions are broad and varied. When reading about them, always make use of what you decide are good ideas from wherever available, and waste minimum energy on the rest.

Overall, I am still pleased with this introductory effort, and recommend it as a primer on wellness issues, principles, and points of view.

The Berkeley Holistic Health Handbook: A Tool for Attaining Wholeness of Body, Mind, and Spirit. Berkeley, CA: And/Or Publishers, 1978.

The Handbook is the closest thing to an encyclopedia on holistic health that exists. It is as comprehensive as could be expected; if your favorite modality or nontraditional therapy is not covered in this book, it must be pretty "far-out." *The Handbook* contains 110 articles organized in five sections (e.g., healing systems, techniques and practices, legal and social issues), plus an appendix containing an annotated bibliography of holistic books and magazines, journals, films, cassettes, and a thorough glossary of terms. *The Handbook,* while credited to the Berkeley Holistic Health Center, is the work of four practitioners of holistic-health disciplines at the Center: Edward Bauman, Armand Brint, Pamela Wright, and Loren Piper. They have produced a watershed document that can help other practitioners avoid reinventing the holistic wheel. They have selected articles to publish in their handbook that support a number of key principles that they (and I) believe are fundamental elements of the emerging approach to medical care known as holistic health:

· Any treatment should expand personal consciousness and help people see themselves and the rest of the world more clearly.
· The process, the caring and open attitude of the healer, are as important as the specific treatment.
· We are all sentient beings who create our own realities.
· We are responsible for our own health, for our relationships, and for the situations in which we find ourselves.
· Nature is an interactive friend; disease can be an opportunity leading to a healthier lifestyle.
· There are many different systems, healers, topics, and styles of holistic medical approaches to illness and disease.

Strengths

The basic strength of *The Handbook,* which makes the production a winner, is the authors' selection of a score of articles that are outstanding and therefore worth the price of admission. In my opinion, the best of the articles are:

· Richard Miles's introduction on humanistic medicine and holistic-health care, which provides a comprehensive overview of the distinguishing characteristics, modalities, and origins of holistic health.
· Judith Lasater's "Yoga: An Ancient Technique for Restoring Health," describing the history and systems of yoga, and the ways in which yoga is used for toning, fitness, relaxation, and health enhancement.
· The section on holistic techniques and practices, particularly the articles on how to choose a practitioner, nutrition, chiropractic, biofeedback, belief systems in relation to disease, subpersonalities within us all and how to deal with the phenomenon, autogenic training, dreams, and meditation and its healing power.
· Charles Garfield's discussion of the impact that work with dying patients has on the well-being of health professionals.
· Bob Kriegel's "A Sport for Everybody."
· Commentaries on the legal issues affecting holistic health.
· All the articles in the final section entitled "Health and the Community."

The value of so many well-chosen articles in one handbook is the opportunity for the reader to expand his awareness of subjects beyond his current interests. You cannot peruse *The Handbook* without appreciating the vast scope of holistic-health issues; the authors go farther than I would and suggest that all of the disciplines described are facets of whole and integrated systems. Perhaps, but either way a lot of imagination went into the choice of articles. In fact, one of the best articles (Tim Scully on nonmedical uses of biofeedback) was written by an inmate of a federal penitentiary!

Weaknesses

The major problem is that the criteria for selecting or omitting was never defined. There does not seem to have been much concern about "bizarre" or "flaky" approaches masquerading as holistic health. Every reader will have his or her own choice of articles that should have been rejected; my choices are the commentaries on health and psychic awareness, healing sounds of a psychic counselor, and inner healing (about the latest in a long chain of "holistic" gurus, faith healer Ruth Carter Stapleton). On the other hand, given the number of issues, techniques, systems, and miscellany thrown into *The Handbook*, the presence of only three schlock entries does not seem a serious shortcoming. And it is worth reemphasizing, what I find void of merit may represent the highlight of the book for you.

Other, lesser objections are that some of the material seems dated; the early editions had no price or address; the drawings with the articles (without the authors' consent or awareness) occasionally do not adequately reflect the content of the materials; and the editor occasionally was out to lunch when certain sentences got published. My favorite example of the latter is in the biofeedback article, as follows: " . . .a British researcher named Richard Caton discovered that the brains of monkeys and rabbits generate electrical signals, which vary with arousal from sleep, death, exposure to flashing lights, and other stimulation." Flashing lights are one thing, but what do you suppose the "other stimulation" might have been to arouse these monkeys and rabbits from death? Whatever — it is a super handbook.

Roberts, Toni M., Tinker, Kathleen, and Kemper, Donald W. *Healthwise Handbook: A Guide to Responsible Health Care.* Garden City, N.Y.: Doubleday, 1979.

Medical self-care, the ability to recognize a wide range of common illnesses and to know how to treat such problems effectively, when to call a health professional, and how to prevent such difficulties in the future are all basic elements of personal responsibility for health. The *Healthwise Handbook* is a consumer guide to this first wellness dimension.

Roberts, Tinker and Kemper (and graduates of their program) have taught self-care classes to thousands of people in recent years, using the model described in this book. Unlike almost all other self-care authors, these writers do not overlook the forest of a wellness lifestyle for the trees of playing doctor on yourself.

It is not possible to read this book without appreciating the all-encompassing ethic of assuming primary responsibility for your own health and pursuing a wellness lifestyle. These values alone recommend the *Healthwise Handbook*, but there is much more. By understanding the basics of self-care for such problems as backaches, headaches, injuries, emergencies, skin disorders, colds and other respiratory conditions, you are in a better position to make wise medical as well as health decisions. The handbook is complete without being dull; the writing style is informal and clear, with plentiful illustrations and easy-to-comprehend examples.

Strengths

The handbook fully details all five wellness dimensions (though the category names are a bit different) and emphasizes that self-care is the beginning of a wellness lifestyle, not an end in itself. I found the chapters on nutrition and exercise to be well-integrated with the other materials, and the discussion of mental wellness (i.e., environmental sensitivity) the highlight of the book.

Throughout each section, you are reminded of the importance of "whole-person" health care — that there is usually more to a symptom than meets the eye, or than is giving you pain. Other characteristics of the handbook that I appreciate are the inclusion of interesting tidbits (e.g., more people die annually as a result of bee stings than from snake bites), and the recognition that belief and will power are key ingredients in the healing process (e.g., the observation regarding home treatment of warts that "faith and incantations" are as effective as faith and over-the-counter drugs).

Weaknesses

Not very much remains to be desired. The *Handbook* covers just about anything you might want to know in order to treat (or avoid) common illnesses and potential medical situations. The major hazard of self-care books is that you can become a hypochondriac reading about the symptoms of all those worseness slings and arrows to which the body is allegedly heir. At times, I think the authors of the *Handbook* go too far in encouraging diagnostic efforts when the time required for such clinical-type efforts could be better devoted to exercise or other health-enhancing activity. An example of this is the suggestion at the opening of the book that you should plan to complete a thorough home physical on each family member twice a year! Unless there are health problems of an unusual nature, or unless you find that small children enjoy the process, and that it widens their curiosity about their bodies and good health practices, such a ritual could be an unnecessary new form of "navel gazing." I also think there is too much of a casual attitude fostered around the drug issue. The chapter on maintaining a home health center reads as if we all need our own personal pharmacy and supermarket of doctor tools.

Well, who needs perfection? — and besides, you are not required to swallow these materials whole. This is a good one — no wonder *Medical Self Care Magazine* called it the best of the self-care genre.

Sobel, David Stuart, and Hornbacher, Faith Louise. *An Everyday Guide To Your Health.* New York: Grossman, 1973.

An Everyday Guide To Your Health is a self-care book with a total emphasis on maintaining and improving health rather than diagnosing and treating illness. The content is based on the techniques attributed to Hygeia, daughter of the ancient Greek god of healing, Asclepius. Hygeia was big on lifestyle, according to Sobel and Hornbacher, coming out long ago for such ideas as a "sound mind in a sound body," living wisely and moderately, health as a natural way of life, and personal responsibility for health. Hygeia's techniques included attention to all the dimensions of wellness, plus a few other specific areas not described in my own wellness books: eyes, feet, hair and skin, tooth care, breathing, laughter, body rhythms, and inner-body/mind work are examples. *An Everyday Guide To Your Health* is organized to continue in Hygeian spirit this work begun long ago.

Strengths

Sobel and Hornbacher have produced a thorough and enjoyable manual on positive health. It is nicely illustrated, sprinkled with unusual but always fitting parables and quotations, and the text is handwritten by one of the authors. In *An Everyday Guide To Your Health,* you will learn much that is of value but not usually available in such a health-enhancing context. This includes excellent chapters on creating a physically supportive environment (clothes, room colors, sounds, reminder signs), tooth care, laughter, and all the other topics listed before. The conversational tone, the humor throughout and the chapters on nutrition and relaxation are added strengths.

Weaknesses

There are scarcely any. There is not much to the exercise chapter (discussed under the heading of body movement); a few of the topics may seem a bit risqué (e.g. "swinging"); and the publications listed for further information are good but a bit dated.

Overall, a fine book.

Vickery, Donald M. *Lifeplan For Your Health.* Reading, MA: Addison-Wesley, 1978.

Lifeplan For Your Health is organized to motivate you to take responsibility for your own health. Vickery describes ways to increase life expectancy and avoid major diseases by helping you recognize disabling medical myths, know what affects health, make wise medical decisions, assess current health risks, and take stock of your lifestyle and the factors which affect it.

It is unlikely that you would be fooled by the medical myths that Vickery defines as beliefs we were raised with, exposed to, or affected by. However, the discussion of the myths is one of the prime contributions of *Lifeplan For Your Health.* It is not common to read a physician's account of the limits of medicine that is so optimistic regarding your power, and pessimistic (or reality-oriented) concerning the relative helplessness of medical science. Vickery's myths include beliefs that health mostly depends on good medical care (I know you do not believe this), that only doctors can tell if you are healthy, that you must see a doctor as soon as a problem develops, that good doctors almost always make correct diagnoses immediately, that a regular checkup or physical is important, that medicine has a cure for everything that ails you. Each of these myths is discussed and debunked at length. Vickery believes that only three routine procedures are justified by the evidence: blood pressure, self-examination, and physical examination of the breast or pap smears. The author suggests that you belong to a small and select group if you do not believe in these myths. Congratulations.

In tracing the limits of medicine, Vickery gives the lie to such pufferies as "the miracles of modern medicine have given us the longest life expectancy the world has ever known." To the author, this is "pure junk," and it ignores the facts of life expectancy. Vickery's analysis of changes in the death rates and periods of major health advances leads to the conclusion that lifestyle is the key health determinant. Therefore, as far as health is concerned, we are on our own in the grip of our habits. While this conclusion is hardly original, it is accurate and stated convincingly. For added interest, *Lifeplan For Your Health* also includes Vickery's laws ("You never get something for nothing; and nothing is 100 percent"), information on the placebo effect, and medical care as a double-edged sword that can save or cost you your life.

Only a few screening tests, X-rays, surgical procedures, and drugs are clearly worthwhile, writes the author, who approvingly reproduces a "prayer" by Sir Robert Hutchinson from a children's ward in a British hospital:

> From inability to let well enough alone,
> From too much zeal for the new
> And contempt for what is old,
> For putting knowledge before wisdom,
> Science before art, and cleverness before common sense,
> From treating patients as cases,
> And from making the cure of the disease more
> Grievous than the endurance of the same,
> Good Lord, deliver us.

Other features of *Lifeplan For Your Health* include a self-scoring assessment system; a quiz to assess your life expectancy and the prospects of your baby's chances for well-being and sections on exercise, diet, smoking, and a long list of other hazardous (drugs, accidents) and disease states. Finally, there is a concluding section on health records.

Strengths

This book belongs at the top of the honor roll list for the four introductory chapters in section one alone. Vickery's debunking of widely-shared medical myths, his critique of lifestyle as the key determinant of health, and his commentaries on cause and effect, placebos, and the limits/hazards of drugs and medical procedures are well worth the price of the book.

Equally potent, though brief, is Vickery's assessment of the power of environmental factors to overwhelm lifestyle. What makes this section so worthy is the author's ability to convey images of awesome forces with the potential to "recreate the Middle Ages." Technology is portrayed as capable of providing some solutions in the short run but likely to create even more severe technological problems in the longer term. Eventually, problems arise for which there is no answer; thus, our future health depends more on learning to use less, to conserve, to recycle, and to throw less away or else we too shall be discarded. The ultimate test, claims Vickery, is our ability to control population, the single best predictor of ill health in the past and the most auspicious indicator of what we can expect of the future.

At times, Vickery is witty, clever, and persuasive as, for example, when he discusses smoking. A balanced discussion, he writes, would require some recognition of the positive side of smoking. That is, the jobs it provides for tobacco farmers and others (seldom mentioned), including morticians, doctors, respiratory therapists, and a host of disease and death workers. As to the argument that antismoking efforts could lead to a loss of jobs and, therefore, is not good public policy, Vickery points out that, by this reasoning, the Mafia should also receive public subsidies. After all, it does a fine job of keeping people gainfully employed and off the welfare rolls.

Weaknesses

The sections mentioned above are so good that the mediocre, dull, and incomplete sections on diet, exercise, mental health, and lifestyle in general are as conspicuous as they are disappointing. Perhaps it is not fair to expect the same level of innovation and thoroughness in every section — why hold the good doctor to such a standard? No good reason to do so — the book's a bargain for the "limits-of-medicine" section alone. Consider the rest filler, especially the last third of the book which details all you never wanted to know or ask about disease-after-disease, *ad nauseam*. Other minor quibbles I have with *Lifeplan For Your Health* include the author's too frequent promotion of his "HEP" (Health Evaluation and Planning) program; a risk-assessment point system as dreary as Cooper's aerobics "by-the-numbers" regimens; overreliance on the dated Holmes stress scale (one stress event is a mortgage over $10,000; how many mortgaged homeowners owe *less* than $10,000?); a statement that, for mental health, we have to settle for a goal of avoiding illness; and excessive attention to varieties of mental illnesses reflective of the overall tendency to dwell upon disease and disability conditions.

Despite the shortcomings, *Lifeplan For Your Health* could help you avoid dangerous tendencies to overrely on doctors and pills, or to under-value your own powers to become far healthier than not sick.

Wildavsky, Aaron *Doing Better and Feeling Worse: Health in the United States. Daedalus: Journal of the American Academy of Arts and Sciences.* Cambridge, MA, Winter, 1977.

This book is an appraisal of the health-care system in the late 1970s through the lens of the leading "establishment"-type power brokers and reformers. Everything you might want to know about the medicalization of health, the technology of medicine, moral issues in therapeutic choice, the quest for medical knowledge, health financing, power centers and decision making, the medical needs of children, institutional change, and much more is all here. What holds together the nineteen separate articles by these titans of health-care delivery are the introductory and title pieces by John Knowles and Aaron Wildavsky. The former provides the historical context, identifies the reasons for the development in the U.S. of an acute, curative case for assuming principal responsibility for your own health; the latter provides the title piece which, in itself, justifies the cost of the entire production and the time required to read this extensive collection of papers.

Strengths

The discussions by Wildavsky and Knowles are truly classics. Wildavsky's title piece is almost as entertaining as it is profound. He writes that the "great equation" is that medical care equals health and, to go with this fallacious equation, a series of equally arresting paradoxes, principles, axioms, identities, and laws. Among my favorites are the following:

· The paradox of time — past successes lead to future failures, meaning that as formerly disabling infectious diseases are overcome, an older population develops and their problems are harder for medical care to affect. Success lies in the past, maybe the future, but never the present.

· The principle of goal displacement — any objective that cannot be realized will be discarded for one that can be at least approximated. In this case, Wildavsky means that process tends to become the purpose — a trap that often catches health planners. In the example given by the author, "health" gives way to "equal access" as the goal of the health system.

· The axiom of inequality — any attempt to make things equal in one area decreases equality in another. You cannot have it both ways — medical care must cost time or money.

· The medical uncertainty principle — there is always another medical approach to be tried (another drug, consultation, or treatment method).

· The law of medical money — the costs of medical care rise to equal the total of all subsidies public and private.

There are other principles, laws, and so forth, but this gives you an idea of Wildavsky's wit as well as his grasp of the issues regarding medical misorganization and misplaced emphasis. He concludes by lamenting our government's propensity to pay both coming and going — once for urging people to assume greater responsibility for their own health and again for their medical bills when the advice is disregarded.

Wildavsky's article is joined by others of considerable merit from a wellness perspective, particularly the discussions by John Knowles and Renie Fox. The former contributes both an introduction to the volume and a learned discourse on the nature of self-responsibility, which both identifies and clarifies the complexities involved in the realization of this first wellness dimension; the latter expands upon the theme of the "medicalization" of health as an indicator of how society deals with issues of value and belief.

Weaknesses

The Winter issue of *Daedalus* is not widely available,* most of the articles accompanying those mentioned above are of modest interest at best, and wellness or health promotion is scarcely treated in any of the pieces, including those by Wildavsky, Knowles, and Fox.

The strengths far outweigh these problems. *Doing Better* is worth the trouble required to secure the volume because of the thoroughness of the three lengthy articles on aspects of self-responsibility.

Nutritional Awareness

Deutsch, Ronald M. *The Family Guide to Better Food and Better Health.* New York: Bantam, 1973.

One of the most comprehensive nutrition books on the honor roll, *The Family Guide to Better Food and Better Health* provides copious breadth and detail on food and health. The emphasis throughout is upon the issues which most confuse the American public — issues which

---

*For information on this issue, write The American Academy of Arts and Sciences, 165 Allandale Street, Jamaica Plain Station, Boston, MA 02130.

the author claims are largely caused by misinformation, deception, ignorance, and frauds perpetrated by health-food merchants and a variety of other "faddists." The tone of the book is set in the foreword, wherein the director of the A.M.A.'s foods-and-nutrition department divides the country into two kinds of people: those who try to learn more about nutrition, and those who retreat into "fads, cults, and unusual regimens, such as vegetarianism." Deutsch carries the attack for another 500 pages, supplying an enormous number of research-finding summaries, quotations from food-establishment sources, personal opinions, and data along the way. Major chapters are devoted to an assessment of what you know and how well you eat, food and life processes, the dynamics of fat and weight, supermarkets and nutritional quality, kitchen safety *re* food poisoning, medical knowledge about nutrition and disease, and food factors in growth and aging.

The Family Guide to Better Food and Better Health contains plentiful charts and tables, illustrations and an appendix on the food composition and nutritive values of nearly anything you ever will consume. In addition, Deutsch has reproduced a recommended- and a *not-recommended*-reading list compiled by a local nutrition association.

Strengths

As the contents suggest, this is an in-depth look at the major nutritional issues of concern and interest. The connection between nutritional awareness and physical fitness is well made; the section on "curing overfat" by understanding the dynamics of body fat and lean muscle tissue is surely one of the highlights of the book. Deutsch is well informed about research findings, medical issues, the biochemistry of human nutrition, and how to avoid deficiency illnesses without recourse to highly unusual food regimens. *The Family Guide to Better Food and Better Health* has it all. It is easy to understand why the book is on the required reading list of nearly all professional nutritionists (and physicians who are interested in the subject). No matter your level of current knowledge, you will find this book a superb reference book and a repository of invaluable data.

Weaknesses

The major problem with *The Family Guide* is the repetitous condemnation of so-called "food faddists" and the attendant apotheosis of the medical establishment and organized nutrition associations. Deutsch takes the villain approach to public anxieties about the quality of our food. Enemy number one is the "faddist" who suggests that doctors and nutritionists are not properly safeguarding the national food supply and eating habits. Dr. Frederick Stare is quoted on page after page, along with the AMA, the food industry, and varied professional nutritionists, to the effect that all is well with the American diet — if the "faddists" would simply hold their tongues and "poison pens" (Stare). Deutsch too often seems to be an uncritical defender of the big-business interests and the medical and nutrition establishments. The recommended and not-recommended book lists are terribly dated, as are more than a few of the references in the text. The advice that only doctors and qualified professionals can answer your nutrition questions is absurd on the face of it. Most doctors were not even taught about nutrition in medical schools, and no insights are provided to help the reader distinguish the qualified experts from the self-appointed gurus.

Lansky, Vicki. *The Taming of the C.A.N.D.Y. Monster.* Wayzata, MN: Meadowbrook Press, 1978.

Designed as an alternative to junk foods, *The Taming* is styled as a chatty, cookbook guide to better nutrition. It contains a few hundred recipes mixed with equal portions of chitchat on sugar, salt, and food additives. Lansky provides a glossary of terms which some readers may find humorous. The book is written for parents, not young people. However, it is included in the honor roll because of its value as a transition diet from a serious junk-food addiction to something a little bit better — on the way to serious reforms.

Strengths

The Taming can be read in five minutes or so, has one or two cute phrases (C.A.N.D.Y. means "continuously advertised nutritionally deficient yummies"), and several useful recipes.

Weaknesses

Lansky's book is superficial, corny, and possibly *hazardous* to your health. The recipes are often loaded with sugar (or dangerous substitutes); fake choices are everywhere (e.g., Lansky writes that the recipes are intended to give a range of alternatives, not to earn "a certificate of nutritional purity"); and dessert is implicitly suggested as a reward for kids.

You will never tame the Candy Monster if you take Lansky's advice or recipes seriously. In fact, if you do, the Candy Monster will eat you — and you will get zits, dark circles under your eyes, and hair on your palms.

Dufty, William. *Sugar Blues.* New York: Warner, 1975.

If Lansky's book on *Taming of the C.A.N.D.Y. Monster* represents a toothless capitulation to the sugar beast, this book must be considered a fearsome, all-out nuclear attack designed for complete annihilation and no-quarter-given savagery. The (S.U.G.A.R.) monster, in this publication, gets just what he (or she) deserves — the unrelenting calumny of an angry and usually persuasive author, with a little help from fellow dragon-slayer Gloria Swanson, a natural-foods buff and advocate of nutritional pathways to a wellness lifestyle.

Dufty's personal account of how he kicked the sugar habit introduces the theme heard throughout *Sugar Blues* — that sugar is a destructive addiction of major consequence in just about every disease or plague known to humans, and no doubt the major factor in disasters yet to occur and diseases not even invented. Dufty probably has forgotten more about sugar than you would ever want to know — read this book and you will discover where sugar comes from, what it consists of, how it has evolved, been marketed, studied, defended and attacked. The emphasis, as you might expect, is on the case for avoiding it, and strategies for doing so.

Strengths

If you already know that sugar is about as nutritious as Clorox or Drano, you will love this book. Dufty provides plenty of evidence and entertaining vitriol about a product that truly deserves the attack unleashed upon it. In short, you will find plenty of support for your antisugar bias in *Sugar Blues.*

The best parts of this book for me are the caustic and entertaining writing style (e.g., sugar as an "addictive planetary plague"), the author's interesting personal history, the specifics on why sugar is hazardous to health, the research data, and range of alternatives recommended.

Weaknesses

Even public enemy number one (i.e. refined sugar) tends to get a little sympathy when overkill sets in. On occasion, I think Dufty gets a bit carried away (e.g., when he declares that sugar is not just plain poison, but a poison "more lethal than opium and more dangerous than atomic fallout"). Really, now. Some remarks are dated (*re* Nixon and his Western White House), and others are absurd (e.g., kicking the sugar habit can be lots of fun). Tell that to American teenagers! The major shortcoming is that Dufty ignores the big picture. There's a lot more to nutritional awareness than avoiding sugar (not to belabor the fact that there is more to a healthy lifestyle than nutritional awareness). But, overlook these quibbles — read *Sugar Blues* and you can decapitate the sugar monster.

Gerrard, Don. *One Bowl: A Simple Concept for Controlling Body Weight.* New York: Random House Bookworks, 1974.

One Bowl, despite the subtitle, deals primarily with controlling food attitudes. According to Gerrard, if you fine-tune your mind, emotions, and body perceptions regarding all aspects of the nutritional experience, you will not only lose weight (assuming that is what you want to do for starters), but will enjoy eating a great deal more than you do now.

One Bowl makes the case that food selection and consumption should and can be a fine art. Gerrard wants you to try eating out of one bowl (really!), to do so in separate courses, alone, at home, and whenever you are hungry. His system has five principles: (1) you can lose weight by eating less "disruptive" and more "harmonious" foods; (2) eat whenever you feel hunger and stop immediately when hunger ceases; (3) eat no more than one food per meal; (4) hunt for just the right food for the individual mood you experience at the time of hunger; and (5) become aware of the importance of how food is prepared and the effects it has on your digestive system.

One Bowl will be the smallest and briefest book on your wellness honor roll library shelf: it's 4"x5½" and only fifty-four pages. Yet, Gerrard covers a lot of information on his unique method for satisfying food feelings and promoting inner harmony. Suggestions are offered for choosing a bowl, de-socializing the act of eating, what to do about liquids, snacks, and restaurants, and how to "create yourself" and achieve peace of mind.

Strengths

This little treasure makes a delightful and persuasive case for eating as an important emotional experience. It will help you to tune in to your body, trust in your own food judgments, and become more attuned to body harmonies and free from food dependencies. You will enjoy Gerrard's gentle style and the author's willingness to share his personal experiences in developing and refining the "one bowl" system.

Weaknesses

The one serious problem with this book is that it could be hazardous to the health of readers who are looking for "the magic bullet." The book does not provide a comprehensive understanding of what you should know to pursue wellness. Gerrard fails to acknowledge that there is more to well-being than weight control. Some statements may upset traditional nutritionists (e.g., fat people do not eliminate enough; your body will always act in the most healthy way it can; eat whenever you are hungry, and so forth). Those who are unaware of Gerrard's influence in the overall wellness movement may not appreciate that he is fully committed to the value of exercise and all wellness dimensions. As noted, these shortcomings only apply to the innocents who believe a book must be swallowed whole or not at all, and who therefore might not realize that this approach is most useful as a short-term, partial step to greater food consciousness and body awareness.

Read this book and experience food not only by its taste in your mouth, but also through an "inner body" understanding.

Lasky, Michael S. *The Complete Junk Food Book.* New York: McGraw Hill, 1977.

A benign look at something we are all presumed to be doing because it tastes good, but reluctantly so, because we know it's not good for us: consuming vast quantities of junk food.

Lasky's book brings you more information than you probably knew was available about the psychology of junk food, its health implications, an "almanac" on its varieties, and a rating compendium of national and regional junk favorites. The latter includes the name of product and manufacturer, a list of ingredients, and five measures (sugar and oil quotients, dental rating [e.g., "tooth rotter"], nutrient level, and calorie count). Included are descriptions of how the merchandisers manipulate us and an account of the negative things that await junk-food junkies (zits, tooth decay, malnutrition, diabetes, hypoglycemia, *ad nauseum*).

Junk food is defined as any food that relies on sugar and/or fat as its primary ingredient. Lasky tells us that some junk food is surprisingly nutritious, while taking the position that, since you (and he) are going to eat the stuff anyway, you might as well learn how to select the better quality junk. Thus, the purpose of the book is to help you differentiate "good junk" from glump junk, "gold" from glop.

Strengths

Lasky writes with humor from well-researched notebooks. He proves himself a phrase-maker (e.g., "kiddie litter") and a certified junk-food junkie himself, telling us of his frequent breaks for Hostess

Ding-Dongs and the like. Much of the information is of interest, such as the data on our "nutritional" patterns: 100 pounds of refined sugar consumed per person per year, 55 pounds of fats and oils, 18 pounds of candy, 756 donuts, and so on.

Other notable features include an analysis of common additives in food, a discussion of the psychology of junk-food advertising and consumption, an explanation of the trials and tribulations facing those who try to produce "good" junk, and occasional strong statements about certain horrible products that represent the pits of an already odious commodity. For example, his commentary on Hawaiian Punch by R.J. Reynolds Tobacco conglomerate:

> ... No amount of ethyl maltel (a flavor enhancer) could help this taste. It doesn't even quench your thirst. Food processors call drinks "punch" when they have no definable flavor. If you drink this garbage, someone should "punch" some sense into you.

I especially welcomed Lasky's attack on mom and dad for mindlessly promoting junk-food tendencies by using sweets as reinforcers, and the fact that he is not afraid to name names when slaying dragons. For example, on the claim by the Wrigley Gum people that gum chewing stimulates excess saliva which neutralizes mouth acidity, Lasky notes that any dentist will advise that this is a "crock of spit."

Weaknesses

Despite the title, this is not a complete junk food book. A complete book on junk food would urge you not to eat junk food, which Lasky does not do — despite his own evidence that abstinence is the only sane course of action. The book is an anomaly: it would have you become a discerning buyer of that which a discerning buyer would never buy. He fails to interpret and translate his own data into the one obvious and essential conclusion: Don't eat the goddamned stuff!

Leonard, Jon N.; Hofer, J.L.; and Pritikin, N. *Live Longer Now: The First One Hundred Years of Your Life.* New York: Grosset and Dunlap, 1974.

Live Longer Now is organized as a well-documented brief for a low-fat, high-carbohydrate diet in combination with a moderate exercise program. It is based on the experience of the Longevity Center in Santa Monica, California, where the authors tested their 2-loop-program approach with over 2,000 persons who had suffered heart disease, diabetes, hypertension, arthritis, and other degenerative diseases.

This book has all the studies, data, and research information you would ever want to read on the causes of various chronic diseases. The authors identify in no uncertain terms the hazards of certain "gremlins" — namely, excess fat, sugars, salt, caffeine, and cholesterol. The value of, and recommended approach to, a regular exercise program called "roving" is described, and a detailed strategy for effective food shopping and cooking is outlined.

Strengths

Live Longer Now is good, basic reading on the hazards of low-level worseness. It is, despite the title's emphasis, especially appropriate for young people. It contains data descriptive of ways that the youngster is damaged in the near-term behaviors that culminate in chronic disease in the long term. The link between all the grim disorders of worseness and sedentary, unexamined lifestyles is persuasive — a characteristic of the book that alone makes it worthy reading. You should find useful the analysis of how youngsters get ripped off by the food companies and advertisers, and the suggestions for avoiding such traps and pitfalls.

The strongest sections of the book are the nutrition chapters. Information worth considering regarding protein and amino acids, meat products, processed foods, the role of key nutrients, and various players in the game of health is provided in an understandable, useful format.

One of the authors' more creative efforts is found in the introductory pages in a discourse on the quality of life and the perennial issue of what happens if everybody pursues wellness, therefore adding more "old" people to society's burden. Their response: wellness would extend the "middle years," not the late years (i.e., being 65 would be more like being 45); productivity would be greater; one's range of opportunities would be extended; the burden of "older people" would be lifted from the society; and the population pressures would be minimal relative to reproduction changes in a single generation.

Finally, *Live Longer Now* deserves a special place on your reading list because it offers specific and practical implementation strategies for exercise and nutritional regimes, and because the emphasis for the recommended 2100 Program is on the positive aspects, not just the usual disease avoidance.

Weaknesses

The major problem from a wellness perspective is the complete neglect of dimensions other than the nutritional and fitness areas. The existence of stress is simply acknowledged in the context of a few disease conditions, and even in this context is waved off as inconsequential. Self-responsibility and environmental sensitivity are alluded to indirectly, but scant attention (at best) is given to both. Thus, the 2100 Program is incomplete as a lifestyle approach to well-being. (Curiously, they never do explain why the program is called the 2100 Program.)

As with most health books, the emphasis, regrettably, is predominantly on the horrors of worseness rather than the joys of wellness. More than half the book is on disease avoidance; as with Moses' Ten Commandments (nine of which are "shalt nots"), the authors' five "commandments" for healthy eating are all "don'ts!" There is some attention to the benefits, as noted earlier, but the focus is on living longer by avoiding a host of degenerative diseases. Of course, if this works for you, great. However, efforts over the years to persuade people to "give up" something have not been highly successful. As you know at this point, the orientation from a wellness perspective is to live well for the satisfactions health-enrichment choices bring, not for the gruesomes they forestall.

There are lesser annoyances — the usual deferential attitude toward the medical establishment; the authors' unwillingness to name real brand and product names of companies producing "garbage"; (e.g., "corporation A" and "sugar yums"); and production errors (mailing address is referenced but omitted).

The existence of the Longevity Center and the growing reputation of the authors, in combination with all the attractive features of *Live Longer Now* mentioned above, make the reading of this book well worth your investment in doing so.

Osman, Jack D. *Thin From Within.* Washington, D.C.: Review and Herald Publishing Association, 1981.

Thin From Within is a guidebook, written in a conversational style with a heavy emphasis on personal responsibility, nutrition, and fitness. The author summarizes his main points at the beginning, repeats them at the end, and details them in the middle. You get the message in *Thin From Within*!

The message is that values and beliefs underlie food and activity patterns. It is important to enjoy dining, to eat slowly, to concentrate on the process as an exclusive function when you do eat, to respect the nutrient content of foods, to get plenty of daily activity, and to follow dozens of other sensible, often mentioned, good nutritional practices. All these are important in Osman's program, but *most* consequential is the notion of total health.

Total health to Osman encompasses a holistic philosophy of social, emotional, physical, intellectual, sexual, and spiritual dimensions essential to being fully human, alive, and unique. This philosophy permeates the book.

Thin From Within provides plentiful technical detail about nutrition and fitness, offers charts and tables for reference, and is loaded with checklists and hints for doing all the right things.

Strengths

Osman is on target on all the important issues, in my view. He covers the critical knowledge areas thoroughly, gives little quizzes or questions to ponder after each section, and writes in an understandable, coachlike fashion. In addition, he shows why bariatricians or "fat doctors" could be hazardous to your health (i.e., due to their pill-pushing tendencies), and offers criteria to employ in assessing the costs and benefits of alternative weight-loss and other programs affecting diet and activity.

Weaknesses

Some of Dr. Osman's "thought cards" and "motivational quotes" may strike you (as they did me) as somewhat schlocko or saccharine. Examples abound but three should suffice:

- "If you eat too many sweets, you'll take up two seats!"
- "Emotions are like rain showers — you can get caught in them when you least expect it."
- "You can't push a button for good health, but you can push yourself away from the table."

Purists may be startled to read, "Use artificial sweeteners occasionally if you must use sweeteners at all." Ex-fatties and optimists may be upset to read that "You are never really cured of being overweight," that control of the problem is the best you can hope for. Finally, there may be a few (like myself) who will wish Osman had kept God out of it: the last part of the book is more a religious sermon than a diet and activity guidebook.

Despite these minor flaws, *Thin From Within* is a winner. You can get it by writing to Fat Control, Inc., P.O. Box 10117, Towson, Maryland 21204, $7.00 postpaid.

Mayer, Anne. *Better Food for Public Places: A Guide for Improving Institutional Food.* Emmaus, PA: Rodale Press, 1977.

Better Food documents the abominable state of institutional food practices throughout the U.S., provides a comprehensive accounting of why this situation exists and the harm it does, and makes a case for (and outlines approaches to) more natural foods in schools, hospitals, nursing homes, and other institutions. Mayer argues that places that should serve the best quality of food often serve the worst. Major attention is given to the issues in bringing nutritional changes for children and in feeding the sick and elderly. Of special interest is a blueprint for action in dealing with the vending-machine-revenue monster. Four pioneering success stories are described to illustrate the feasibility and lessons of sound, nutritious institutional feeding, and details are provided for storing natural foods, special equipment requirements, cost-saving methods, and preparation techniques. An appendix listing resources for further information, including books and simpatico manufacturers, completes this one-of-a-kind survey and how-to publication.

Strengths

Read *Better Food* and you will surely pack a lunch if you have to visit someone in a hospital. The chapter on feeding the sick is enough to motivate the reader to stay well at all costs. Food is usually catered by profit-oriented, junk-food purveyors. Nutritious meals to facilitate the patients' return to health are the exception, not the rule. Mayer cites studies that show hospitals as "pockets of malnutrition" where at least five percent of patients suffer hospital-induced malnutrition, and where one-third become anemic during their stay. The strengths of the book are not restricted to dramatic statements of the problem, however. Mayer describes success stories and then outlines how better foods can become the norm in all kinds of public places. No food-service manager should be without this important book. It is clearly written, well researched, and amply documented with good references for additional study.

Weaknesses

None.

Orbach, Susie. *Fat is a Feminist Issue.* New York: Berkeley, 1978.

If you are an obese female, this could be the most important nutritional awareness book on the honor roll; if you are an obese male, this also might be the most important book on the list. In Orbach's psychoanalytic perspective, the greatest factor contributing to obesity is compulsive eating, an individual if unconscious protest by women against sexual inequality. The extensive material, including case studies, an analysis of the meaning of fat/thin/and the hunger experience for compulsive eaters, guidelines for self-help, theories of weight loss, and medical issues all make for valuable reading for males as well as females, both fit and nonfit.

Orbach defines food compulsiveness as eating when not physically hungry, spending a lot of time thinking and worrying about food and fatness, scouring for the latest diets, feeling out of control around food and poorly about yourself because of it, and feeling awful about your body. For at least half of all U.S. women, obesity and overeating have joined sex as central life issues, writes Orbach in the introduction to *Fat is a Feminist Issue.* The author believes that compulsive eating is rooted in the social inequality of women, that getting fat is a purposeful act or challenge to role stereotypes, a way of saying "no" to being without power and, as such, is an adaptation (albeit not a very functional one) by oppressed women.

Orbach, a feminist and psychotherapist, describes seventeen examples of "what it means to be fat" in our culture, the popular conceptions of the experience that result from chronic, compulsive eating. For these and other reasons, the author acknowledges that a woman's desire to be fat is seldom conscious, yet, being so serves several functions. These include space and protection for feelings, escape from the prospects of competition (and inevitable defeat), and the eradication of competitive feelings.

In moving away from fat, Orbach suggests that the unconscious motivation for it (and the compulsive eating that creates it) must first be exposed and understood by the obese person. If obesity is to be discarded, however, something else must be available for that which provided a powerful protective role. Orbach suggests the alternative is to see that the qualities (e.g., protection, strength, mothering, assertion) the obese person attributes to fat are in fact possessed at a deeper and truer level.

Strengths

Fat is a Feminist Issue offers many insights into the fat culture. It is a readable, persuasive analysis from a psychotherapist's perspective, which is not something that is often available from that profession. Orbach's approach to self-awareness and self-help seems sensible and effective, starting with the goal of breaking addictive relationships with food and progressing to more natural and relaxed connections beyond fat to the body and the whole person.

I especially appreciate the emphasis on helping obese women comprehend that fat often serves in strange and harmful ways to create awesome problems. For me, the most valuable lessons of the book are the clarification of feminist aspects of compulsive eating and fat, the connection of self-esteem and eating patterns, the discussion of food addiction and its implications, the guidelines for self-help groups, and the evocative and no-nonsense phrases for the hazards of diets, pills, and surgery (e.g., they represent "technological fixes" for attitude and behavior problems).

Weaknesses

Although Orbach's analysis seems right on target for many obese women, I am less confident that the explanation holds in all female fat cases. After all, there *are* a good number of thin women out there who have not chosen fat as a shield from male aggression. I also suspect that many men are affected by basically similar pressures. For this reason, it would have been good to have another chapter on the relationship of societal expectations on male food compulsion, and subsequent retreats into fat. This could have been included in a single chapter; if Orbach had done so, *Fat is a Feminist Issue* would have been no less interesting to females but a lot more useful and attractive to males. Then again, this may be the subject of the author's next book.

In the next edition, I hope the author writes more about other aspects of a healthy life — beyond getting clear on relationships with men, on the traps of compulsions, on the futility of fat, and other nutritional insights to related and equally vital topics — such as physical fitness, stress awareness and management, and environmental sensitivity.

Till then, there is much to reread and ponder in the current edition. *Fat is a Feminist Issue* is another well-marked book in my wellness library — I suggest it for yours.

Reich, Lawrence. *From Fat to Skinny.* New York: Wydon, 1977.

This is a first-person account of how author Lawrence Reich went from 300 to 162 pounds. It is Reich's way of presenting a "modeling strategy" for learning to change and for becoming the person you want to be. It is not a diet book in the usual sense — it contains no recipes or lists of foods you must or must not eat. It rejects pill remedies and never once urges you to get a doctor's permission before embarking on an individualized program to realize new weight goals. What *From Fat to Skinny* does contain is an outline for getting started on a new eating pattern — a pattern that encompasses thin rather than fat attitudes and habits.

Reich provides a philosophy for learning to be thin. He demonstrates the power in the concept of taking responsibility for your own health, fate and, in particular, body weight. In doing so, the author debunks all the myths that serve as barriers to change (e.g., too old, too dumb to learn new habits) and shows that you are always capable of growing and improving. Reich provides a short course on established learning theory to demonstrate that a thin eating pattern is within your grasp, and organizes the material into twelve "short-cut" approaches for "eating winners."

Strengths

This is a fun book containing a lot of interest for all wellness-oriented diners, whether or not they have a weight problem. The personal approach really works — you come away with a good feeling for the author to go with a sense of power to shape a nutritional-wellness lifestyle. Reich's constant humanization of the material, with examples of how friends, associates, and clients have experienced one lesson or another, adds both interest and credibility. The approaches introduced are really workable — from imaginary eating binges to tape recordings to positive reinforcements to self-rewards to models to trusted others. *From Fat to Skinny* is an adventure — and another tool for building a wellness style of eating.

Weaknesses

Some may find Reich's call for the free-flowing use of the imagination a bit far-out, especially if the reader's use of said imagination has not been exercised a great deal since childhood. Others may find the author a little reckless in the cause of self-determination — such as when he suggests that the French seemed to function as well on a continental breakfast of coffee and a roll as others on a more normal diet. How does he make this startling observation? By traveling with French people in Morocco — and not seeing anyone faint in the streets before lunch!

Ignore this peccadillo — *From Fat to Skinny* is a winner.

Stress Awareness and Management

Bloomfield, Harold H. and Kory, Robert B. *The Holistic Way to Health and Happiness.* New York: Simon and Schuster, 1978.

This book is subtitled "A New Approach to Complete Lifetime Wellness." It's not new or complete, but it does add another important chapter (and a substantive one at that) to the wellness literature. It could have been subtitled "The Transcendental Meditation (TM) Way to Wellness," because so much of the authors' interpretation and counsel are weighted around TM approaches.

Bloomfield and Kory organized this work as a consequence of their belief that the greatest obstacle to health for most people is a lack of knowledge about it. Thus, they provide lengthy sections on the issues they believe readers need to know about in order to lead healthier lifestyles. These include weight reduction, fitness, change strategies, stress management, and ways to overcome a shopping list of high-risk behaviors or conditions which are essentially elements of a low-level worseness lifestyle (smoking, alcohol abuse, depression, chronic fatigue, and so forth).

Strengths

There are many, but the two that stand out in my view are the authors' discussions of a wellness profile (based on the work of Maslow, Sullivan, Adler, and others who were among the few investigators to study healthy people), and their acknowledgment throughout of the ways in which the culture shapes either healthy or worseness behavior norms. Other valuable aspects of *The Holistic Way* are:

- An emphasis on the importance of meeting security needs and raising self-esteem as foundation steps to a wellness lifestyle.
- A restatement and insightful discussion of two basic wellness tenents — that neither Rome nor a wellness lifestyle is a made-in-a-day proposition, and not to "give up" a high-risk behavior until you don't need it anymore.
- An entertaining and thoroughly persuasive case for the cardiovascular, recreational, and ancillary (e.g., cure for insomnia) benefits of guilt-free and joyful sex.
- A take it slowly, enjoy each step of the way attitude as the preferred approach to a wellness lifestyle.
- Imaginative phrasing, such as a reference to an "ardent interpersonal power player."

Other aspects of the wellness approach to an enriched existence which I found well developed and described were the lists of helpful hints after each section heading, the illustrative case discussions, and Bloomfield's and Kory's ability to show persuasively that unattended stress can sap your ability to enjoy and perform in every aspect of life.

Finally, a word or two should be written on behalf of the occasional flashes of humor, my favorite example of which was the suggestion that exercise not only reduces anxiety and improves self-image, but also increases sexual "attunement." The phrase I enjoyed in this regard was to the effect that you have not lived fully "until you have taken a jogger to bed, especially if that jogger is you."

Weaknesses

There are so many that you might think I don't really like this book! I do — just about all of the following critical comments are related to the authors' adoption and subsequent interpretation of the wellness philosophy. As a traditional-health or even as a holistic-health publication, few of these weaknesses would seriously detract from the book. Yet, by wellness standards, there are both major and annoying lesser problems. Let's begin with the major problems.

The first of the major problems is that *The Holistic Way* obscures two of the first tenets of wellness: (1) it reinforces rather than combats the individual's dependence on doctors; and (2) it legitimizes and continues the culture's overemphasis on drugs.

An occasional suggestion that obvious medical problems should be discussed with a physician would be OK, but the authors go overboard with the "... need for you and your doctor to reassess the basis of your health and well-being." *You* need to assess your state of health and map your own wellness program, and you don't need your doctor to do it — with or for you. The doctor is not an equal partner in the design of your wellness lifestyle. He or she may, if clearly warranted, be called upon occasionally to serve a (subordinate) consultant role as ally or facilitator. References in *The Holistic Way* to patients, to "leading physicians" this and "doctor-endorsed" that, are out of sync with the wellness ethic of personal responsibility and accountability. (On another occasion, a wellness lifestyle is called a holistic-health program, further contributing to the medical orientation.) The non-wellness affection for powerful (and other) drugs is seen in periodic supportive references to "anti-depressant medications" (and psychotherapy), as well as advice to use medications as directed, which could be interpreted as "take doctor's orders."

There is an overemphasis on stress management, an understandable situation given the authors' previous publications on TM. Specifically, the benefits and efficacy of the "healing silence" seem overstated. This is promoted as the key to nearly all aspects of a wellness lifestyle — even to the point that it begins to sound like a sort of "magic bullet."

In addition to these serious shortcomings, there are a number of annoyances that detract from the overall impact, among which are the following:

· A section on how to choose a therapist seems totally out of place in a wellness book.
· An overfocus in all parts of *The Holistic Way* upon the manifesta-

tions of low-level worseness (e.g. obesity) to the neglect of a larger framework for dealing with the overall picture (e.g. nutritional awareness).

· A contradiction on an important point. In Chapter 10, you are advised that you do not have to achieve a high level of fitness to enjoy a high level of wellness. In Chapter 23, however, you learn that a prime characteristic of the full well person is a high level of fitness.

· Use of the redundant term "positive wellness." What is wellness if it's not positive? Can you imagine negative wellness? Neutral wellness?

Despite these serious and not-so-serious weaknesses, *The Holistic Way* by my friend Harold Bloomfield and his co-author Robert Kory deserves a reading. It is, on the whole, a fine book and an important addition to the wellness literature.

Davis, Martha, et al. *The Relaxation and Stress Reduction Workbook.* Richmond, CA: New Harbinger Publications, 1980.

The *Workbook* contains a thorough description of the stress phenomenon and the great range of options by which we can adapt to, modify, and profit from it. Twelve different techniques are highlighted for managing stress. Stress concepts are defined, analyzed, and classified, as are environmental, bodily, and psychological stresses.

This is, indeed, a workbook. It is not a list of readings for passive entertainment or intellectual data gathering. It is designed for personal or professional use and abounds with tables, charts, graphs, lists, inventories, and diaries for recall, classification, and self-analysis. You do not read this book — you participate with it.

A unique closing chapter provides a bit of extra counsel and encouragement to those readers who may conclude that the techniques and procedures are too difficult to apply in the "real world."

Strengths

The *Workbook* continually reinforces personal responsibility. The authors rely upon positive payoffs as incentives to learn varied stress-management skills, techniques, and points of view. The most popular excuses for not taking responsibility are skillfully exposed, as are the most common causes for not practicing the recommendations offered. Among the best points made in *The Workbook* are the following:

· That the body registers stress long before the conscious mind lets you know about it.

- That muscle tension is one noticeable body signal to which it is well to pay heed.
- That all your thoughts become reality, and that you are what you think you are — so choose how you want to be.
- That the view you take of any event is more significant than the event itself.
- That the failure to act assertively is a sign that a person does not believe that he/she has a right to a feeling or point of view.
- That culturally implanted "irrational ideas" (e.g., "you need something other or stronger or greater than yourself to rely on") may be at the root of many or most life stresses.

The strongest chapters are those on body awareness, meditation, autogenics, assertiveness training, and refuting irrational ideas. Any three of these would justify reading the book. The presence of five such gems of stress-management erudition and guidance make this a special entry in the wellness bibliography.

Weaknesses

The authors overlooked several opportunities to at least acknowledge that activity in certain other dimensions (e.g., physical fitness) would have beneficial consequences on a person's ability to deal with upsets and difficulties. The ending seems weak, with its concern about or anticipation of failure. A number of typographical errors are excusable, but one illustration is not. In a "coping skills" discussion, Davis and company list numerous thoughts for the preparation, action, fear, and congratulatory stages of stress events and circumstances. The authors suggest that you make a list of coping statements meaningful to you, and that you keep them in handy places. So far, so good. But guess where one of the "handy" place illustrations is? You may not believe this, but here is what they wrote: "Slip them inside the cellophane of your cigarettes."

Just for the record, be advised that smoking is not a very wise mechanism for coping with stress.

Despite this ridiculous illustration, *The Workbook* is a fine publication, and I recommend it.

Gawain, Shakti. *Creative Visualization.* Mill Valley, CA: Whatever Publishing, 1978.

Creative Visualization is defined as "the technique of using your imagination to create what you want in your life." Everyone uses visualization; unfortunately, in doing so we seldom are creative about it. Gawain suggests, in fact, that cultures set us up for negative imaginings that build and reinforce a sense of lack, limitation, difficulties, and problems as our lot in life. *Creative Visualization* is written to train you to use a positive-oriented, conscious imagination to reverse these tendencies. With these methods, Gawain believes you can create love, fulfillment, health, satisfying relationships, and other desired states of being.

Gawain first describes how *Creative Visualization* works, then follows the discussions with practical exercises. Major attention is given to relaxation, affirmation, prosperity programming, giving, healing, and meditation. Several techniques are dramatized; goal setting is encouraged and explained; and a variety of processes for health and beauty are recommended.

A considerable emphasis is given to the value of discovering your higher purpose or area of contribution to the world. This is seen as a part of being a well person in the larger sense of the word.

Books and tapes are listed for further reading and study.

Strengths

Gawain offers us a gentle, peaceful, and prosperous view of life. This book conveys a genuine concern for others, and the techniques point the way to the use of stress management for peak moments of human experience.

Creative Visualization is filled with good ideas and practical techniques and processes for raised self-esteem, one of the foundations of a healthy person. The visualizations are imaginative and the commentaries on health and illness make a lot of sense. Wellness-oriented nutritionists will approve of the eating rituals; others may find special uses for Gawain's goal-achievement technique called "treasure-mapping."

Finally, extensive affirmations are included. These give added credibility to the practicality and creative challenge which self-hypnotic suggestions can represent in shaping a wellness lifestyle. A sampling of my favorites might be of interest:

"I love myself completely as I am, and I'm getting better all the time."
"I'm glad I was born and I love being alive."
"I deserve love and sexual pleasure."
"The more I love myself the more I love _____."

Weaknesses

Creative Visualization suffers from a number of problems endemic with "new-age," "holistic"-type publications. At times, readers may feel uneasy with such phrases as "the healing energy of the Universe," unless they have taken something like Leo Sunshine's "prosperity training," from which a lot of the material is taken. More serious is the concern that too much faith may be invested in too few approaches to optimal health. In the present case, this means overreliance on multiple forms of creative visualization to the neglect of action in the physical world. Affirmations, no matter how deeply felt and often practiced, will not make you fit and trim. (In fairness, Gawain would not suggest otherwise, but some readers may miss the subtle message that mental preparation leads to, but never substitutes for, peak performance.)

Overall, make no mistake. This book is a good one. I recommend it highly.

Pelletier, Kenneth R. *Mind As Healer, Mind As Slayer: A Holistic Approach to Preventing Stress Disorders.* New York: Delta, 1977.

Mind As Healer is a comprehensive and scholarly account of psycho-physiological events regarding the body's response to stress. Special attention is devoted to the mind-body link, the role of consciousness, and the applications of techniques such as biofeedback, meditation, and autogenic training. Stress conditions and responses are categorized and shown to be clearly linked with illness conditions, with the focus on the primary afflictions of civilization. Case histories and research summaries are generously employed to support the conclusions offered, and a provocative final chapter describes the philosophical foundations of holistic medicine. An extensive bibliography of books and journal articles is included.

Strengths

The highest use of this book could be as a required-reading assignment by doctors to their clients on the occasion of a first visit for psychosomatic illness — which includes nearly all visits. The second highest use would be as required reading for doctors. It may encourage those who treat symptoms with drugs to think about underlying phenomena, in this case, stress and the maladaptive ways that most of their clients respond to it. Among the sections that I considered of special value were the following:

- The reinterpretation of the term "psychosomatic" as characteristic of all disorders, in that mind and body are always involved in disease etiology or causation.
- The view of symptoms as an early indication of excessive mind-body strain.
- The defense of the placebo effect and the importance of marshaling its powers and subtleties for healing purposes (rather than

continue the current pejorative, "put-down" usage of "only" imaginary value).

· The discussion and promotion of the holistic-health model, particularly the concluding chapter wherein Pelletier notes six characteristics of holistic medicine.
· The explicit recognition that a great limitation of the healing professions today is an overemphasis on pathology and disease relative to a massive unawareness of health and health enrichment.
Given the nature of current disease, this is properly termed
"dangerously short-sighted."
· The emphasis throughout all chapters on the importance of gaining personal control and self-responsibility for healing and positive health.

Weaknesses

As a thorough and authoritative description of the dynamics,
sources, and effects of stress and approaches for raising stress awareness and management skills, this work leaves little to be desired. Only
one problem got in the way for me. While other dimensions are recognized in the first and last chapters, I felt that many opportunities were
lost to reemphasize the value of an integrated stress response. This
excessive reliance on mind techniques (biofeedback, visualization, autogenic training, and meditation) seemed most apparent in the chapters on stress diseases and methods of controlling stress. In both cases,
the influence of nutrition, exercise, and purpose-in-life factors deserved greater mention. A lesser problem was the overall orientation,
which seemed a bit too heavy on illness and disease and light on health
maintenance and wellness.

A fine publication — one of the best on the stress dimension.

Schafer, Walt. *Stress, Distress and Growth.* Davis, CA: International
Dialogue Press, 1978.

Stress, Distress and Growth contains a detailed exposition of the
theme that stress is inevitable and desirable, and that our ways of
dealing with it determine our results for better or worse. Major sections
are devoted to the nature of stress phenomena (the basics, as discussed in Day Nine), on social forces which precipitate stress overloads
in the unprepared, and assorted strategies for coping with and exploiting stress events and circumstances. The foreword includes a nice bles-
sing by the godfather of stress management, Hans Selye. Footnotes,
bibliography, index, and a generous variety of illustrations and figures
are included.

Strengths

The book introduces a lot of new concepts and refined techniques for managing stress. The focus is on harnessing stress for the achievement of personal goals, not just the avoidance of illness conditions. The chapter on the relationship between stress management and running is excellent, as is the discussion about the social nature of stress, particularly at the workplace. Fortunately, detailed strategies are suggested in each circumstance, and they do seem plausible and practical.

Weaknesses

Stress, Distress and Growth does what the author set out to do, but some of the material is a bit dated (Holmes's Life Change Index). The style is somewhat dull, though no problems of any consequence were noted.

Shealy, Norman C. *90 Days to Self-Health.* New York: Bantam, 1978.

This book is promoted as a 90-day health program, but it is in fact a treatise on the importance of maintaining health on a lifetime basis. The emphasis is on relaxation, exercise, body control, balance, and other elements of wellness. Shealy terms his program of regular routines for body, mind, and spirit attunement, "biogenics." The goal is harmony of, not control over, the mind (as the author believes characterizes other relaxation-centered disciplines such as Transcendental Meditation and hypnosis). About 80% of the material covers the stress dimension, which is the foundation of Shealy's biogenics program. Much of the book is devoted to mental programs designed to help people stabilize their autonomic nervous system and "tune in to the universal life force." Other chapters treat such issues as pain (its causes, therapy, and management) and varied health-care-system topics (surgery, drugs, hospitalization, etc.).

Shealy is representative of the growing number of holistic-oriented physicians willing to seize the "teachable moment." The illness situation is a time when people can be motivated to look beyond physical symptoms to underlying lifestyle factors. Shealy's self-help philosophy centers on autogenic, affirmative mind, body, and spirit training; and his program of biogenics is the model used at the Pain Rehabilitation Center in Wisconsin, which the author founded and directs.

You cannot read this book without appreciating certain fundamentals of a wellness lifestyle, including an understanding of the extent to which there is no effective alternative to personal responsibility for advanced levels of well-being. You may or may not be comfortable with the biogenics program; you will almost surely be reinforced by, and interested in, the author's ideas on nutrition, fitness, relaxation, habit regulation, and much more.

Strengths

Shealy has a persuasive, low-key attitude that conveys a gentle and caring perspective to his points of view. I like it when he writes that each of us has a spiritual side that is loving and kind, that our goal can be to always direct our thoughts to our highest selves. True health, Shealy emphasizes, results in the long run from integration of body, mind, and spirit aspects of our existence.

If you enjoy drills or self-help exercises, you will find much to work with in *90 Days to Self-Health* — nearly half of the book is given to illustrative techniques. The chapter on emotions and health is surely one of the better descriptions of the issues and self-awareness skills needed for effectiveness in this dimension. Shealy has included excerpts from other contributions, some of which add a lot to certain discussions. My favorite example of this is a skillful relaxation and meditation story by Thomas Elbert Clemmons, a fable involving galactic travel in time and space and a grand cast of characters (e.g., Galileo, Marcus Aurelius, Von Braun, Teller, Robert E. Lee, Einstein, and the "Great Spirit"!).

Weaknesses

The major wellness-related problems with *90 Days to Self-Help* are those common with physician-authored health books. These include, despite the holistic orientation and other admirable characteristics, the following grievances:

- An excessive discussion of illness conditions in the first third of the book (e.g., Shealy lists and describes nine disease classes).
- An overemphasis on reliance upon doctor's permission and clearance before abandoning drugs, undertaking self-health steps, and experimenting with medical self-care.
- A tendency to be too deferential to doctors (e.g., "Do not, of course, stop taking any drug without your physician's advice.").
- The occasional dumb remark, such as Shealy's statement that he "does not believe in divorce" because those who remarry are, in his opinion, no happier. Then, he adds, "Of course, there are exceptions, but my view is not important anyway." As one who falls into the exception category, I wonder why he wrote that line, since he did not think much of his view on the subject in any event. (Furthermore, there *are* alternatives to marrying again or staying in an unhappy union.) In short, I think Shealy fails to

show how this personal bias translates to his point that you should control stress by accepting what you cannot alter and changing what you can.

· Questionable nutritional recommendations, such as advice to eat freely of meats such as lamb, pork, and beef (huge saturated fat content), go lightly on fruits, and consume substantial vitamin pills and bran daily.

Essentially, Shealy is trying to persuade you that what is going on in your mind has more to do with the quality of your body than modern medicine has realized. His book is a valuable record of current understanding and technologies that exist for achieving higher levels of well-being through building varieties of autogenic, mind-mastering, and self-fulfilling affirmative skills. In this regard, it is an important contribution and deserves a reading.

Tanner, Ogden. *Stress.* New York: Time-Life Books, 1976.

This book consists of easy-to-read photographic essays about stress. *Stress* provides just about all you could want to know about the subject — what stress is, what it does, and how it works for and against you. Unlike any other book on the honor roll, *Stress* is best examined in a library, given the expensive nature of this encyclopedic volume and its nonavailability in bookstores.

Tanner provides a thorough review of the development of knowledge about the stress phenomenon. Included are discussions about the role of pioneer investigators (e.g., Johnson, Cannon, Selye), the impact of ubanization (particularly overcrowding, noise, and the threats of rapid change and crime), and the stress-induced hazards of varied life crises.

Other chapters deal with stress-management customs in different countries, ways that the pain (and stress) of grief is managed at times of death, and learning how to cope. *Stress* contains 171 photographs and an extensive bibliography of readings on the subject.

Strengths

Stress contains a good deal of information not generally available elsewhere, and a fascinating collection of documentary photographs illustrating the main ideas in each section of the book. Some of the vignettes are outstanding (e.g., Outward Bound, Parachutists, and the French Resistance Movement), the explanations are clear, and the research documentation is useful for any serious investigator of the stress phenomenon.

Weaknesses

Some sections are silly and poorly done (the worst is about a ranch girl from Oklahoma seeking an acting career in New York); however, the most serious weakness is the omission of specific advice or guidance concerning what to do about stress.

A useful book worth your perusal — in a public library.

Physical Fitness

Anderson, Bob. *Stretching.* Fullerton, CA: 1975.

Anderson's book is a *must* for "stretch freaks," and others (including yours truly) who would benefit from regular stretching if it were enjoyable and shown to be a vital adjunct to any fitness routine. *Stretching* does both: the author has compiled the complete book of stretching and demonstrated how important and satisfying an appropriate routine can be. Anderson maintains that stretching leads to an "opening of the mind" and improved attitudes toward the physical-fitness dimension. In short, an appreciation of this physical art helps any individual, concerned with his or her own cardiovascular level of excellence, to better integrate fitness with other aspects of the full life.

Stretching is described as the foundation for fitness. It can help you relax, experience physical and psychological revitalization, enable you to avoid or minimize injuries, increase your flexibility, and develop your potentials, as well as your patience. Anderson focuses on such basics as when to stretch (anytime and as often as you feel like it and always before and after vigorous physical activity), and who should stretch (everyone, naturally). Chapters are devoted to specialized stretches for specific major sports and, after describing the basis for the epidemic proportion of low-back problems in the U.S., on proper back care. However, most of the book describes how to stretch. Anderson uses the phrase "the developmental stretch" as the essence of the activity; this is midway between an easy and a drastic stretch. The developmental stretch is one element; the other phases of proper and optimal stretching are rhythmic breathing, a noncompetitive attitude, and pain avoidance. There are enough exercise routines described and illustrated to keep you stretching for a lifetime (fifty-eight major-muscle-group routines are covered).

Anderson confirms what a lot of young people have suspected: that some schools give fitness or physical education a bad rep or negative connotation by inadvertently making it seem a punishment, drudgery, bore, or otherwise "unfun" affair. This happens when the subject is "taught" or managed by uninterested or unqualified people, when it is an "add-on" topic for rainy days, or when it is simply omitted or neglected for whatever reasons. *Stretching* begins with an incisive analysis of the unhappy results of this benign neglect — the health losses attributed to a nation of spectators.

Strengths

Anderson makes stretching seem practical and enjoyable, as well as essential, for a balanced fitness routine. His book is easy reading and can be used as a reference manual while practicing different stretches. I appreciate his ability and insight in the manner of linking stretching with movement, fitness, relaxation, and nutritional awareness. I particularly admire his creative commentary on physical stretching and the powers of the mind — such as in penetrating old barriers and psychological "hang-ups." In short, Anderson shows that regular and skillfull stretching helps us better perceive our personal potentials. Throughout this lengthy book, Anderson reminds us that we are all unique beings, and applies this understanding to the discussions of all the principal stretch routines. The emphasis is on finding our own comfortable and enjoyable rhythms — when stretching and in other things we do.

One other special strength is a section written especially for coaches and teachers. The philosophy noted above is well capsuled in this commentary and is recommended reading before going ahead with the stretch routines.

Weaknesses

It sounds good to me, but some readers may be a little skeptical of Anderson's statement that an inflexible body is less open to new undertakings in the larger sense of living and conducting one's affairs. It may be so, but it does sound a bit facile. The only serious omission, given what the work attempts, is the absence of reference to a substantial body of data which supports the beneficial claims for stretching. Anderson must believe the benefits are too obvious and self-evident — some may not agree. On the whole, a special work of value for the person who wants to be totally fit.

Bailey, Covert. *Fit or Fat.* Houghton-Mifflin, 1978.

Covert Bailey writes about ways to lose excess fat (not weight) while gaining optimal fitness. Along the way, he describes myths about fat people, why diets don't work, how to choose an aerobic exercise, sensible food patterns, and a lot more.

Strengths

Fit or Fat is clear, entertaining, and informative. I got so enthused reading it that I wanted to exercise immediately — which was inconvenient since I was in a hot tub at the time. (I settled for vigorously fanning my girlfriend with peacock feathers.) Bailey does know his subject — he runs a clinic, leads seminars, and conducts fitness testing. His experience shows throughout the work. I got the impression that, if he could, Bailey would send your muscles to school to learn how to burn calories. Save the tuition and read the book — it's all there.

I especially liked the sections on "spot reducing" (forget it, you are just "tenderizing" fat — you need aerobic or whole-body exercises) and the distinction between work and exercise.

On a technical level, you will learn how muscle cells burn glucose, the hazards of a high-protein weight-loss diet, and the dynamics of fat conversion. But, most important, you will find the motivation for adequate daily exercise if you do not already have it and reinforcement for your current lifestyle if you do. Can't beat that.

Weaknesses

There are not many. Bailey could have addressed some other areas (how to avoid overuse of doctors, the hazards of junk food, how to build support groups, etc.), but apparently this was not his intent. He claims that women are, because of 30 percent greater fat composition than men, winning 50- and 100-mile runs. Where? As a runner and reader of the runner publications, I have not heard of a single win yet by a female in competition with men. I would love to see it, but I do not believe it has happened — so far. (A recent chat with the author revealed that what he intended to write was that the performance gap is narrowing.) These are peccadillos — you should enjoy this book as well as benefit from it.

Burger, Robert E. *Jogger's Catalog.* New York: M. Evans and Co., 1978.

Jogger's Catalog contains most of what is worth knowing concerning this most popular form of exercise. In addition to basic data that every runner knows or ought to, Burger provides photos, opinions, anecdotes, book reviews, race profiles, runner sketches, and resource lists (podiatrists, newsletters, etc.). Lengthy sections are devoted to what running does for your head, tests and diets to keep you running well, foot care, running techniques and apparel, clubs and races to join, running tours, unusual running events, and how to keep a personal exercise log.

Strengths

This book is dynamite if you like running. The photos and stories make *Jogger's Catalog* as timely and interesting as your favorite monthly running magazine, but the serious chapters and references add a deeper quality of new learning for most readers. It is, as the author attempted, a *Whole Earth Catalog* for runners.

Weaknesses

Few, given the purposes of the book. A little recognition of what runners should know about nutrition would have made *Jogger's Catalog* a better source book. Naturally, some recognition of the value of running as a first step toward a healthier, more satisfying "whole-person" lifestyle (i.e., wellness) would have been terrific as a component of this book. Still, it is the best of the running books to date, in my view.

Cooper, Kenneth H. *The New Aerobics.* New York: Bantam, 1970.

Another in the aerobics series by the author (and his wife), this edition provides detailed charts on age-adjusted exercise programs. The book is a guideline or data-reference source — there are more tables, charts, and tests than commentary. *The New Aerobics* contains an extensive introduction on the impact of the aerobics system, a description of the elements of "required" physical examinations, fitness-test categories, tips and safeguards, and points of view regarding exercise for women and indoor conditioning. Cooper adds a section on questions most often raised during his aerobics lectures and a time-based point system for walking and running in tenths-of-a-mile increments.

Strengths

Cooper lends credibility to assertions about the value of exercise, which a lot of people apparently need from a doctor-authority figure. *The New Aerobics*, as with the other aerobics books, presents the white-coated physician with the stethoscope and chart-pad image giving "permission" to the patient to exercise without overdoing it. As mentioned, a lot of people, mostly older, sedentary Americans, will respond to this paternalistic approach. For them, this characteristic of the Cooper aerobics system is a strength. Another is the reference value of the extensive data assembled on the value of varied exercise routines.

Weaknesses

What is a strength to some may be a turn-off to others. For me, the "by-the-numbers, get your doctor's permission" philosophy is a turn-off. The Cooper approach does not encourage self-responsibility and personal independence, exercise as play or fun, and an understanding of the interrelatedness of fitness to all the other wellness dimensions. *The New Aerobics* (and the "old aerobics" by this writer) is to your fitness potential what the concept of health is to the average person, namely, a conservative perception far short of what could be, given higher standards and goals toward excellence.

Farquhar, John W. *The American Way of Life Need Not Be Hazardous to Your Health.* New York: Norton, 1978.

This is a comprehensive and well-documented text on the importance of individual lifestyle for health and well-being. The author is a physician who has personal experience in working with large numbers of people toward the goal of developing effective methods for achieving self-directed change in key wellness areas. Specifically, Farquhar is the director of the Stanford Heart Disease Prevention Program, a large-scale research endeavor set up to explore the medical, social, and psychological issues related to the prevention of cardiovascular disease.

The American Way opens with a dramatic account of a friend's heart attack. Farquhar describes the setting, symptoms, and medical wizardry applied for revival and treatment, postoperative strategies and costs, months of agonized efforts at recovery and, despite it all, the friend's premature demise. The little drama well illustrates Farquhar's primary point: that this nation wastes vast sums of money and other resources on the dying to the unconscionable neglect of the living. According to the good doctor, 90 percent of strokes and heart attacks are preventable. *The American Way* is organized to show how to do just that: major portions are devoted to stress, fitness, nutrition, the development of worseness lifestyle patterns, and ways to reduce weight and stop smoking. In addition, a chapter is devoted to methods for achieving self-directed lifestyle change, and the techniques described are illustrated in each of the major subject-area chapters (e.g., exercise and stress management). For the research-oriented and readers interested in additional sources, a useful reader's guide is included.

Strengths

This is one of the better books available on the importance of lifestyle. The greatest strengths of *The American Way* are:

- The emphasis on an integrated lifestyle for pursuing your highest potentials for well-being.
- The insights and data contained in the chapter on "stress and how to cope with it."
- The clear linkage between your behavior in one dimension and your effectiveness in the other dimensions.
- The laying-to-rest of protein and calcium-requirement myths, which Farquhar shows to be vastly exaggerated in our culture.
- The "tools" described for use in self-directed change, especially contingency contracting, daily-activity logs, self-contracts, internal monologues, notebooks, booster sessions, tapering, and behavior rehearsal.
- The willingness of the author to express himself forthrightly (e.g., connecting white bread with vitamin-B deficiencies, cigarettes as having an even greater impact on heart attacks than on lung cancer), and picturing Americans as leading the world in the percent of population that is overweight.
- The optimistic "you can change if you want to" attitude — so long as you prepare yourself with the right tools (provided), and sufficient time (bring your own — and don't rush it).

I enjoyed Farquhar's style — he is readable, not dogmatic, pushy, or self-aggrandizing. I especially appreciated his perspective on cultural change as a vital element in personal reform. At one point, he even postulates that times will be better when the healthy minority becomes the majority culture. When that happens, the culture will automatically reinforce health-promotive behaviors (e.g., real food in schools, stress-management training on the job) and discourage disease-producing norms (e.g., allowing smokers to foul airline cabins, tolerating junk food in hospitals). Thus, the benefits of good living will, as Farquhar suggests, be easier for all to achieve.

Finally, special mention must be given to the superb section on stress awareness and management. Farquhar persuasively charts the impact of unattended stress and shows how it is the most influential factor in cardiovascular disease. He demonstrates that mastery of this wellness dimension enables advances in other dimensions, especially exercise, eating habits, and smoking neurosis. The six stages of Farquhar's stress-management change program are: (1) to identify the stress problems; (2) build confidence and a commitment to change; (3) increase awareness of stress sources and responses; (4) develop a stress-management-action plan; (5) evaluate the plan; and (6) maintain regular stress-reduction practices. If you only read this section, you would learn a lot about deep muscle relaxation, mental relaxation, and vis-ualization — which alone would be worth the purchase price.

Weaknesses

When a very good wellness book has weaknesses, the flaws seem more noticeable than would be the case in an average health-related publication. *The American Way* has a good number of miscellaneous shortcomings, and a couple that are serious.

The minor problems include:

· An overemphasis on disease avoidance to the neglect of health enrichment.
· Excessive mention of Stanford personalities and studies — out of balance in relation to the paucity of other references in the text.
· Cartoon drawings that distract and which, in my view, are sloppy, unfunny, unsubtle, and sophomoric.
· A few too many diaries and contracts to keep anyone motivated to do all that Farquhar recommends.
· The exercise chapter is weak, in my view, with too much of a focus on Cooper's boring aerobics program and too little attention to exercise other than walking.
· Some of his expectations of the reader seem impractical — such as expecting periodic rescoring of varied risk levels every six months for at least three years:

The serious problems with Farquhar's good book are:

· A tendency (no doubt unintended) to "give permission" for, or to at least legitimize, one or more deadly worseness habits ("limit" alcohol to not more than ten percent of total calorie intake and maintain a caffeine habit or "no more than" four cups a day).
· The usual medical overprotectiveness customary in health books, especially when authored by physicians.
· The total neglect of two vital dimensions of wellness: namely, self-responsibility and environmental sensitivity (by whatever name — the issues involved in developing these lifestyle skills are simply ignored).

The strengths far outweigh the shortcomings. Farquhar has written an important and good book.

Fixx, James F. *The Complete Book of Running.* New York: Random House, 1977.

As the title suggests, if you are interested in nearly all phases of the running phenomenon, you have come to the right place. Fixx's purposes are to "change your life" and to tell you nearly everything you could reasonably want to know before — or after — embarking on a running approach to physical fitness. The book describes Fixx's (and others') views on *why* to run (physical and mental effects, longevity, benefit comparisons with other sports), *how* to run (from preparation to Boston, kids to the over-forty set, heart patients to Bill Rodgers, and more), and interesting events and characters in the "world of running " (running publications, philosophers, scientists, and fanatics).

Fixx paints a clear picture of how sick the "normal standard of health" truly is, how unhealthy most medical doctors are, and how optimum conditioning can be pursued on a lifetime basis (i.e., by devoting a portion of your existence to jogging/running).

Strengths

- The book stayed on the best-seller lists nearly forever — in no small part due to the fact that it is interesting, personalized, and loaded with valuable information for anyone even remotely interested in running, runners, or both.
- The resource guide (bibliography) at the end of the book is useful to the serious student of running.
- The author is guilty of extensive name dropping — which adds rather than detracts from the messages being conveyed. It really *is* of interest to learn what the superstars and other notable characters told Fixx relative to diet, running, benefits, styles, practices, and so forth.
- *The Complete Book of Running* is likely to encourage and guide a great many people in the art and sport of running. Who would not be attracted to the myriad benefits — increased oxygen capacity and overall endurance, greater heart-pumping power and muscle strength, and added lung capacity, for starters. The best, however, may be the psychological goodies — the joy and subtle "highs" runners experience.
- The section on "kids" running is brief and weak, but the fact that a chapter is devoted to young people who run is a definite plus.
- Other highlights which I consider the strengths of the book include Fixx's willingness to be critical (e.g., his "on-target" criticisms of "cosmetic health clubs" which encourage little or no

cardiovascular exercise), his discussion of nutrition for runners, and his emphasis throughout on the uniqueness of each runner.

Weaknesses

- As is typical of all magic-bullet books (i.e., x or y or z is the one true way to total well-being), *The Complete Book of Running* contains excessive claims (will "change your life," make you healthier, happier than you ever imagined you could be, etc.). It seems that ex-fatties are the worst offenders in this regard. Fixx tells us that he was a beefy 213¾ on November 25, 1968.
- Occasionally, the author throws out a statistic that is wildly speculative and attempts to cloak it with scientific respectability. For example, women marathoners have been dramatically getting faster in the past ten years, a progress which Fixx traces by citing time improvements in the women's world record. So far, so good. He then notes that "it was recently estimated on the basis of scientific analysis" that a woman will someday run a 2:23 marathon. In the few years since that was written, several women have come very close (i.e., 2:25 and 2:26 have been run by three different women), and it is just a matter of time before large numbers of women begin to realize their true capabilities in all sports. "Scientific analysis" also could be used to demonstrate that, since 95% of all passengers involved in fatal air crashes ate carrots within two weeks of the disasters which befell them, carrot eating is therefore hazardous to your health. The point is that it is not always necessary to cloak a reasonable point of view or opinion in analytical mumbo-jumbo. It certainly is not required to predict a 2:23 woman marathon.

Despite these annoyances and the overexposure of the author in ads for sugary cereals, credit cards, pop, and what-have-you, the book is a useful introduction for those getting started on a running program. It is much better than the new version.

Fluegelman, Andrew ed. *The New Games Book.* Garden City, N.Y.: Headlands Press/Dolphin/Doubleday, 1976.

The theme for all sixty new games presented by the editor and the New Games Foundation is "play hard, play fair, and nobody hurt." Common to all the games is the idea that there are no spectators, second-stringers, or losers. The new games are for the whole person who wants fun with his or her fitness. The games described, which of course are even more fun to experience than to read about, are designed for two to two hundred, are available for all ages and sexes, and are well illustrated with hundreds of expressive photos.

The introductory chapters of *New Games* describe how the concept of new games came to be (it began with World War IV!), as well as how to "playfully" organize and referee such "non-contests," and how to stage-manage successful new-games tournaments. Essays by Stewart Brand, Bernie DeKoven, and George Leonard add yet another dimension to this complete book for the whole, fit, and well player of the new games.

Strengths

The strongest point of the book is that you get the sense early on in your reading of *New Games* that the activities described truly are vigorous and enjoyable. In short, the book inspires you to go out and play and have fun — what more could anyone want of a publication? Play a new game today, and tomorrow you will find it easier to pursue an older game for cardiovascular excellence, flexibility, and strength.

In addition, *New Games* is a pleasure to read. It helps you think beyond games to new and more satisfying ways to live. New games are great for winners and also for people with an underdeveloped sense of humor. The situations *New Games* create help us to laugh at ourselves in a knowing, kindly, and forgiving way. Steward Brand describes how he deliberately created games that would give participants a chance to get in touch with joy, cooperation, and the physical side of their being. The result of his efforts are well described in the game of "Earth Ball."

In one of the first trials of the game, played with a six-foot diameter rubberized canvas, painted with continents, clouds, oceans, etc., and placed in the middle of a football-sized field, Brand announced: "There are two kinds of people in the world: those who wish to push the Earth over the row of flags at that end of the field, and those who want to push it over the fence at the other end. Go to it." Naturally, people charged the ball and began pushing toward one end or the other. At first, one side was clearly dominant, but soon an interesting thing happened which, according to Brand, suggests that some people "can't stand to be on the overdog team." As the ball approached a goal, players from the winning side defected to bolster the force about to be vanquished. And the game went on for hours. Brand suggests that this is a characteristic of Earth Ball — perhaps players just don't want the game to end. So, you can sense from this case what it is like to play new games — the value is in the process, not the outcome.

Weaknesses

Hardly any. A few of the games are a little difficult to understand by reading the rules — sometimes you just have to play to get a feel for the activity. Maybe an instructor should come with the book!

Really, *New Games* is a good book, and new games are lots of fun. I highly recommend both.

Kuntzleman, Charles T. *Activetics.* New York: Wyden, 1978.

Activetics is a popularized fitness program oriented to weight loss. The program has been used for years in YMCAs with much success. It is based on the simple notion that what you take in (calories) and what you burn up (exercise) must be in balance. By controlling these two variables, you can lose or gain what you wish. Unlike aerobics, which concentrates on fitness and endurance, Kuntzleman emphasizes that activetics is focused on weight. Activetics is broader than aerobics, as defined and popularized by Cooper, in that a larger number (unlimited, in fact) of activities are encouraged.

The great obesity problem is not caused by overeating, says the author, but rather "underdoing" or exercising too little. *Activetics* provides a thorough review of important nutritional issues, such as why diet alone is dangerous, why a few extra calories are important, and why people get fat. Included are reviews of popular weight theories (appestat, psychological, and conspiratorial glands), diets (low-carbo, low-fat, low-protein), and gadgets (rubber suits, saunas, belts, machines). Chapters on the activetics program are illustrated with case histories and a lengthy (nearly half the book!) appendix on the caloric values of various foods.

Strengths

The best features of *Activetics* are that it is easy to read and highly sensible. People ought to know these fundamentals about exercise and bizarre weight-loss plans. Kuntzleman does a fine job of explaining the exercise program, and hundreds of ways to burn calories throughout the day.

Weaknesses

The *Activetics* program seems a little oversold. It is most appropriate for those who do not enjoy, or at least practice, serious cardiovascular conditioning on a daily basis. Furthermore, there is a lot more to be gained from exercise than weight control, which is the overriding goal of activetics. The flimsy cardboard "caliper" or "fitness finder" and the explanation given for its use does not seem practical or accurate; it would be better to encourage readers to have a body-composition test done by a professional.

A good book with solid content.

Mirkin, Gabe, and Hoffman, Marshall. *The Sportsmedicine Book.* Boston: Little, Brown, and Co., 1978.

Want to know more about the biochemistry of fitness and nutrition, principles for avoiding and/or caring for athletic injuries, training methods, and the relationship between exercise and sex? Mirkin and Hoffman have written a "how-to" guide that explains what science knows and several hundred of the world's greatest athletes, coaches, and trainers in nearly every sport believe about these and other issues related to serious exercise. Fifteen sportsmedicine myths are analyzed and debunked — e.g., fit in just minutes per week, there's no need to stretch if you are fit, vitamin supplements improve fitness, athletes need more protein, salt tablets should be taken. The rewards of exercise are made explicit; the working of muscles and universal training rules are explained; and commentaries on vitamins, minerals, common injuries, and finding a sportsmedicine-oriented physician are provided.

The Sportsmedicine Book contains a step-by-step program for running and a nationwide listing of names and addresses of sportsmedicine doctors, podiatrists, and clinics where stress electrocardiograms are available to the public. The book is loaded with informative tables, charts, and illustrations, and the 8½" x 11" paperback size makes it convenient for reference purposes.

Strengths

The essential value of *The Sportsmedicine Book* is that it is filled with interesting, important information on vital fitness issues. Another strength is that all the material is presented in understandable language with references to the experiences of well-known athletes and coaches. The chapters on exercise myths, nutrition, and injury avoidance and treatment provided the substantive highlights for me. In visits to fitness centers in different areas of the country, I have observed fitness directors making reference to Mirkin's and Hoffman's book. The use of *The Sportsmedicine Book* as an authoritative source seems well justified.

Weaknesses

Except for quoting the opinions of a lot of sports figures and their own knowledge, which is undoubtedly substantial, there is surprisingly little research evidence cited in this reference book. In fact, there is no bibliography or listing of citations to be found anywhere in *The Sportsmedicine Book.* In my view, given the authors' purposes in providing a "how-to" work on basic principles, this seems a major flaw. A lesser problem is that a few of the quotations from sports luminaries are silly, and would better have been omitted, especially in the fluff chapter on sex and sport.

Sheehan, George. *Dr. Sheehan on Running.* Mountain View, CA: World, 1975.

Dr. Sheehan is considered by some the Shakespeare of writer-runners. The short pieces on varied aspects of running are taken from his columns in *Runner's World* magazine and the *Red Bank (N.J.) Register.* The essays address issues beyond the limited focus implied by the title: Sheehan uses running as a metaphor for living life to the fullest and enlarging your existence. Running, or becoming and staying fit, is equated with a positive self-image. Your body is judged a mirror of your soul and mind, and youthfulness is maintained by your level of conditioning. Exercise, in sum, is considered to be the best "high" available — and legally, at that. By developing our physical capabilities to the maximum, says Sheehan, we discover our spiritual and intellectual potentials.

Strengths

You cannot read this book and not recognize the rewards of a wellness lifestyle, among them being greater levels of joy in life, energy and vitality. Fitness is properly depicted as fun, and play as the key to well-being and the best defense against the absurdities of everyday life.

The "abnormality" of our standards of normality is described — by this Sheehan means that "true normal" is the condition of the well-conditioned athlete whose body functions at maximum efficiency. We can all operate at this level if we so choose.

I enjoyed the literary aspect of the articles — and Sheehan's debunking of the medical imperialism surrounding physical exams and stress testing.

The sterility of Cooper's "aerobics" is justly panned — with a comment that Cooper's point system measures everything except why people exercise and enjoy pursuing their own well-being. Unlike all the aerobics books, Sheehan's work provides motivation because of an emphasis on the positive side of the wellness equation.

The most important strength is Sheehan's emphasis on self-responsibility — never better expressed than in his recognition that health, as with excellence in any endeavor, is best derived from our own efforts.

Weaknesses

Just a few complaints, and each relates to an imbalance in Sheehan's approach to fitness to the neglect of other dimensions. Specifically, he gives too little attention to nutrition (knocking vitamin supplementation in the process) and stress management (regrettably, he even OK's, or resigns himself and the reader, to coffee and aspirin). In addition, his statement that "a world without runners would be unlivable" seems somewhat exaggerated.

Nevertheless, *Dr. Sheehan on Running* is superb reading — I recommend it heartily. *Sheehan on Running* is better, in fact, than his several more recent (and expensive) titles.

Smith, David. *The East/West Exercise Book.* New York: McGraw-Hill, 1976.

There is more to fitness than cardiovascular endurance exercises, as David Smith shows in this popular book on fitness from a multicultural perspective. The disciplines described and illustrated by a male (the author) and a female model derive from ancient as well as modern practices, from Oriental and European as well as American forms. While especially suitable for young people, all exercises are applicable to the not-young as well.

The East/West Exercise Book is divided into five parts: the first section deals with the author's purposes, the value of "free-and-easy" body movement, the joining of East and West (e.g., yoga, Kung Fu, Arica, mime, and heart-rate monitoring), and "harmony" technique (centering, relaxation, grounding, and proper breathing); the second part concerns five separate cycles of exercises involving nearly 100 different routines for overall or total-body fitness; the third part introduces games for "freedom" as well as fitness, plus exercises for school, home, or office; the fourth part provides help or advice, and special movements and postures for problem areas; and the fifth part contains food for thought (the author's nutritional-awareness program) and a description of alternative East/West pathways to healing and staying well in the first place.

Strengths

Smith's book is an original, and so is he (of course, we are all originals, but this fact is a bit more pronounced or noticeable in the author's case). The man has *done* everything he writes about and seems to live the whole-person philosophy that comes through in all parts of the book. *The East/West Exercise Book* is super for reading about interesting possibilities to supplement your aerobic exercise in order to gain added flexibility, coordination, balance, strength, and agility — and to have fun in the process. There is none of the win-lose mentality in

Smith's approach — everybody wins by trying and enjoying. The themes heard throughout are cooperation, courtesy, sportsmanship (sportspersonship?), self-reliance, self-responsibility, emotional maturity, and individuality.

Some of the games, exercises, positions, and techniques are simply terrific. They are both fun and helpful for conditioning purposes. One of my favorites is nude dance, but don't overlook paddleball, being an animal, bioenergetics, and all the others. Many will, no doubt, appeal to you. I suspect you will also relate well to Smith's nutritional viewpoints, which are very similar to the wellness-oriented food practices recommended at most wellness centers.

One of the reasons I feel good about these exercises and Smith's philosophy is the soft-sell approach used throughout.

How many times have you read books and articles by and for runners, for example, that provide in-kind suggestions for dealing with hecklers (e.g., jog over their car hoods, throw rocks, copy license plates, try twenty-seven proven put-down wisecracks, and so forth)? Smith urges a different psychological ploy — to smile at the occasional heckler or say something positive, such as "I wish I were you" — none of which is likely to make the heckler any less miserable in the long run, but the short-term effects on you are superb.

Weaknesses

The suggestions regarding other systems of healing are incomplete and, in some cases, pretty far-out. Furtheremore, Smith acknowledges this "hard-to-handle" aspect, yet, goes on to urge that you consult your physician before attempting any of the alternative methods or health systems. Surely he must realize that most Western-trained doctors would not respond favorably to cleansing processes ("Kriyas"), reflexology, Tibetan eye charts, and fasting.

An outstanding fitness book, and useful in at least three other dimensions, also.

DeVries, Herbert A. *Health Science: A Positive Approach.* Santa Monica, CA: Goodyear, 1979.

This is the first textbook to orient material to the perspective of positive health, and thereby avoid the major criticism directed toward health educators (i.e., that they are doomsaysers and "warriors against pleasure"). DeVries traces the history of science, medicine, and health in the introductory pages, and concludes that the current generations have a better shot at control over their own well-being than their counterparts at any time in the past. His book is designed to help young people and others make the most of their opportunities by clarifying the choices to be made. By focusing on self-responsibility as the key to positive outcomes rather than just disease avoidance, DeVries opens up subject areas not usually addressed in health-education textbooks.

Health Science: A Positive Approach is organized into nineteen chapters and five basic parts; only the first and last address positive health. These sections contain detailed discussion and review of pertinent research data on fitness, stress, and exercise dimensions, as well as information on weight control, muscle and joint health, and positive mental well-being (environmental sensitivity). Other areas discussed include negative high-risk behaviors and hazards (e.g. chronic fatigue, drug and alcohol abuse, infectious and degenerative-disease avoidance, and smoking); factors largely outside of our control but important to understand (e.g., heredity, aging, and sickness); preventable situations (i.e., accidents); and sexuality, marriage and family. Each chapter ends with a summary of the most important points discussed, as well as references and recommended readings.

Strengths

The sections on cardiovascular fitness and muscle strength are the most thorough and helpful parts of this good book. This is not unexpected, since the author is a distinguished scientist in the field of physical education and exercise physiology. Whether describing ways that exercise can improve your health, the pulse-rated system of monitoring heart-rate intensity, the nature of aerobic activity, or the health hazards of sedentary lifestyles, DeVries is on solid and convincing ground. The summaries, tables, charts, and references to research findings likewise contribute to learner involvement and comprehension of the material.

The highest strength of *Health Science*, however, is the fact that DeVries recognizes, and throughout every chapter reinforces, three fundamental notions of a wellness lifestyle: (1) that positive, health-enrichment approaches and inducements are better than negative, fear tactics; (2) that people are unique and individualistic, and must be encouraged to find their own approaches to effective lifestyles; and (3) that optimal well-being requires an integrated program — DeVries covers all five dimensions and more.

Weaknesses

There are very few, and only one weakness is of major consequence. Some chapters seem to warm up to the topic and then drop it, providing teaser information but nothing really new on the subject (particularly evident in the concluding chapter, "Marriage and the Family"). DeVries apparently has never heard of holistic health, wellness, or any of the hundred or so forms of alternative approaches to dealing with health problems other than physicians and related healers. The chapter entitled "Finding Appropriate Medical Services" is simply illustrative of an old-fashioned and narrow outlook on what the health-care system is or could be. This is the only major flaw of the book.

A superb item for your wellness library.

Eisenberg, Arlene, and Eisenberg, Howard. *Alive and Well: Decisions in Health.* New York: McGraw-Hill, 1979.

Alive and Well is a conservative but thorough medical self-care medical-awareness textbook focused on the myriad ways to minimize illness risks by taking responsibility for your own health. The emphasis is on prevention principles, basic health facts, state-of-the-art developments, and the basics of self- (and medical) treatment. Organized into twenty-six chapters (with appendices, glossary and bibliography), the Eisenbergs' book is focused on six overall themes: (1) learning to cope with life — or the search for identity, maturity, change, and the dynamics of mental health; (2) illness prevention and staying well in the first place — on effective use of the medical system, fitness, nutrition, and other issues in taking care of yourself; (3) disease as the other end of the spectrum — on the basics of body responses and the gamut of ills to which flesh is heir (infectious diseases, coronary, cancer, and other degenerative maladies; trauma, and the appropriate role of surgery and other approaches); (4) drugs and consumers — on the use and misuses of the medicine chest, alcohol, marijuana, and so on; (5) love and the life cycle — on human sexuality, courtship, family planning, pregnancy, childbirth, parenting, and aging; and (6) the business of health — on the health-care establishment, ethical issues, and heroes and quacks.

Strengths

Alive and Well is the product of the authors' extensive review of journals, books, and files, supplemented by interviews and a clever synthesis of disparate items from scattered sources. The basic attraction of this book is that it is encyclopedic and timely. The organization of the material works; it is easy reading without being simplistic in presenting subtleties with facts, and controversies with state-of-the-art beliefs. *Alive and Well* is a thorough consciousness raiser. The fact that it is loaded with photos, poems, cartoons, illustrations, quotes and chapter-ending summaries of key points, simply adds to the value of what the Eisenbergs have produced. Who, for example, will not appreciate a little humor, such as the following quote buried in a learned discussion of the anatomy of human sexuality: "Mark Twain once said that Niagara Falls was the second biggest disappointment to honeymooners."

Weaknesses

I would have liked a greater emphasis on the nature of positive health (e.g., characteristics of superhealth people), ways to create supportive environments for wellness, and recognition of the trend toward and value of the wellness movement. A more critical appraisal of medical practices and the medical establishment also would have been appropriate, in my view.

Greening, Tom and Hobson, Dick. *Instant Relief: The Encyclopedia of Self-Help*. Wideview Books, 1979.

Instant Relief is about mitigating problems through psychological self-help. It offers a sense of direction that reduces dependence on experts, and increases reliance on oneself. It is to emotional/mental health what medical self-care is to physical health — a guide to being your own doctor, most of the time. *Instant Relief* is not about the pursuit of optimal functioning, though much of the material is useful for these larger purposes.

Greening and Hobson use a five-part approach to just about whatever does or could upset you. This method involves: (1) deepening your insight into the dynamics of the problem; (2) identifying unconscious payoffs which holding on to the problem provide; (3) acknowledging your responsibility for making changes; (4) becoming aware of new ways of thinking, feeling, and acting; and (5) abandoning the mediocrity of avoiding illness in favor of pursuing growth and self-actualization (wellness).

An index is provided, as is a guide to assessing the need for professional help (emphasis on the limits of same) and how to manage and profit most from such relationships.

Strengths

Instant Relief drives stakes through the hearts of disabling myths and draining dependencies. They focus on our inherent powers to relearn ways to interpret events and circumstances, and on psychological techniques that are crucial for getting free of "situational prisons" and beyond the neutral point of not being ill. (Illness in this case is represented by a supermarket list of 100 possible maladies or upsets.)

The advice on all 100 issues is consistently sound. You can benefit from this opus even if you are experiencing none of the difficulties discussed in this little encyclopedia of upsets.

Greening and Hobson deserve special recognition for moving the counseling function (regarding mental and emotional difficulties) away from the goal of not suffering, to one of making paths to optimal functioning. They cite a variation of Freud's remark on the purposes of psychoanalysis (to effect or change deep, disabling neuroses for the ordinary neuroses of daily life), and emphasize the inadequacy of this limiting point of view.

The greatest strength is the fact that the counsel on nearly every problem is thorough, sensible, and consistent with the promise and payoff of self-empowerment. Other highlights include good quotes ("Do you think that sex is dirty?" Woody Allen: "It is if you're doing it right"), and references for further study presented at the conclusion of each topic.

Weaknesses

Hardly any. Naturally, everyone will find some of the included items of no interest whatsoever. I wish they had discussed poor food habits, sedentary lifestyles, and low-level-worseness environments, but that is just nitpicking.

A superb handbook for do-it-yourself mental health, and a valuable reference when specific information is needed about specific problem areas. *Instant Relief*, while not a quick fix for anything, does contain nearly 400 small-type pages of socko information. A winner from A (abortion) to W (writer's block).

McCoy, Kathy, and Wibbelsman, Charles. *The Teenage Body Book.* New York: Pocket Books, 1978.

This book is much like *Our Bodies, Ourselves*, the landmark publication on medical self-care for women, with the focus in this case on young people. It is comprehensive in scope, covering nearly every imaginable topic of interest and many not found in standard self-care books. Major topics are — growth concerns common to young women and to young men, feelings, nutrition, exercise, health habits, mental well-being, illnesses, sexuality, venereal disease, birth control, parenthood, and appropriate medical care.

The format of *The Teenage Body Book* is to present a series of questions asked by young adults on the topic of each of the fourteen chapters. The questions are followed by a general discussion and specific answers to each query. The book is well illustrated, easy to read, and loaded with useful counsel regarding problems and issues that come up for nearly every young person.

The appendix contains a detailed resource guide for young people interested in getting help. Addresses of low- or no-cost clinics and birth-control facilities catering to adolescents are provided. Also included are addresses of crisis centers, hotlines, run-away switchboards by state, and a wide range of other resources, including books and films especially applicable to youth.

Strengths

The true value of this book is found in the authors' forthright, sensible, caring, and understandable responses to questions posed by young people, and in the discussion of basic issues in each chapter. I found the sections on nutrition, exercise, sexuality, birth control and feelings especially outstanding. *The Teenage Body Book* is holistic in the best sense of the word, in that the whole young person — mind, body, and spirit — is addressed. It is easy to read and should be part of every young person's library.

Weaknesses

As expected when one of the two authors is a physician, the usual medical conservatism is evident in some sections. While self-responsibility is acknowledged as the key to a full, healthy, and happy life, there are occasions in the text when greater autonomy from the medical system could be encouraged.

Highly recommended.

Spino, Dyveke. *New Age Training for Fitness and Health.* New York: Grove Press, 1979.

New Age Training for Fitness and Health is part autobiography, part advertisement for the services and achievements of the author, and part "New Age" pep talk. "New Age" methods, words, and techniques are introduced by the score in discussions of alternative approaches to total health or wellness, with the focus on nutrition and physical fitness. Major emphasis is placed upon lengthy testimonials by Spino's clients; names of prominent healers and holistic places are dropped liberally.

The thesis of *New Age Training for Fitness and Health* is that a holistic movement is underway which will enable a "New Age" of spiritual and psychic awakening or consciousness, that the movement is represented by such approaches as Ms. Spino advocates and practices, and that everyone who tries such methods will evolve and transcend and thus become a "New Age" person — and maybe a "New Age" coach!

Chapters are devoted to self-assessment questionnaires, processes for change and strengthening the will, body movement, the "feminine principle" and masculine problems, nutrition, flexibility, male and female training for the "New Age," and "graduate" training for same. All sections are filled with case histories, or more accurately, client commentaries, on the wondrous transformations evoked by the "New Age" coach and author.

A final chapter contains an outline of Spino's vision of an ideal center, which she hopes someday will come about in order to further advance the era of the "New Age." The book includes a short listing of references, films, and tapes (sold by the author), as well as many photos of Ms. Spino and her clients.

Strengths

New Age Training for Fitness and Health is an original — the language, the hype, the concepts, and the claims are all designed to "ignite," to motivate, and to inspire. There are no doubt many readers, perhaps yourself, who will let go and revel in the psychobabble of the "New Age," enjoy this book immensely, and profit from it. For that reason, it is an honor roll selection — different strokes can attract varied folks into a wellness lifestyle. Jargon aside, Spino is definitely providing another pathway to wellness — and her methods often do work. (I retained Dyveke on two occasions to work with middle-aged, sedentary health planners — and sure enough — she succeeded in activating characters who had given up on fitness as teenagers.)

This book should be read while playing Mozart's *Jupiter* Symphony with candles aglow, incense burning, fireplace crackling, and all the rest — the mood must prepare you for a leap of faith. Spino is never dull, her perspectives are highly unusual, and her ability to evoke images is well-developed (e.g., "energy streamers," "sensing," "inner space"). On occasion she is profound, as when composing thoughts for the gods while buffeted by unknown creatures during a long sea swim:

> "Dear Beautiful, Living Things of the Ocean, please forgive my intrusion into your territory. I mean you no harm and I know you mean me no harm. Yet I am human and my flesh is soft, so please, Dear Universe, protect me in my swim and guide me."

If you are open to and ready for all the "far out" concepts, characters, and language of the "New Age," you have come to the right place — Spino will help you play the edges of your consciousness.

Weaknesses

Personally, I must not be ready for the "New Age." This book evoked my gag reflex throughout. I have my doubts about the "New Age" as it is herein described — it just seems awfully flaky to me. I have difficulties getting beyond the "old age" when I encounter phrases such as "prana at the apex"; the predominance of references to psychics, clairvoyants, mystics, and readers, and what I found to be gross male/female stereotypes. The organization of the material is confusing, wishful thinking gets passed off as current trends, and inaccuracies call all the material into question (Spino misspells my name, improperly references my book, confuses my association with Dr. John Travis, and incorrectly claims that I have been her student). On at least one occasion, Spino is totally inconsistent. She writes on page 250 (and elsewhere) not to be indiscriminate or to be seduced into following anyone yet, yet on another page (191) you are instructed to follow *her* procedures "to the letter." Come on, Spino, you can't have it both ways. Finally, I think the book is grossly overpriced at $12.50.

Overall, this book is of interest *if* you are inclined to see things from the author's "New Age"-colored glasses.

Environmental Sensitivity

Allen, Robert F. (with Charlotte Kraft). *Beat the System: A Way to Create More Human Environments.* New York: McGraw-Hill, 1980.

Beat the System is about norms, change, freedom, and self-actualization. It presents a systematic process for the humanistic design of cultures that work. It applies to families, friendships, corporations, and all other institutions, such as hospitals and wellness centers. This is a training manual filled with tested concepts and illustrated guides for applying "Normative Systems" in varied settings. It is, more than any book published to date, directly pertinent to the focus of environmental sensitivity in a wellness context. It is a design plan for establishing the kinds of cultures needed to sustain the pursuit of optimal health and whole-person well-being.

Allen and Kraft describe how it is that the norms of all the cultures of which we are a part shape us, for better or (as is more often the case) for worse. The "culture trap" phenomenon is detailed, and just as you begin to think that it is time to abandon all hope, they let us in on the glad tidings: it does not have to be that way.

The alternatives are described in the second part of the book entitled, appropriately enough, "Changing Things." The normative system is presented, along with diverse instruments for understanding prevailing patterns and working with others to manage and secure full involvement in the change process. Four case histories of success are sketched, as is one instance wherein the process failed. Of course, lessons are drawn from both.

Beat the System can be read as a self-help manual, as a kit for organizational development, or as an interesting description of how cultures work. The authors provide generous examples of applicable forms, quizzes, listings, drawings, references, and (were all this not sufficient) pertinent and often profound quotations from varied great thinkers past and present.

Strengths

You cannot read this book and remain unattentive to the basic assumptions of the many subcultures that are central to your health and prospects for success at commitments to a well-being lifestyle. Dysfunctional traditions, fashions, and laws — all have the effect of creating "ceilings on the mind," which the wellness-oriented reader will surely want to raise once such constrictions are noted. The great strength of this book is in the description of the issues followed by real-world cases. The fact that each case is described in accordance with the previously discussed principles for effective norm identification and reshaping adds a skillful element of drama as well as a frame for learning. It should be mentioned that this technique is workable in large measure because the principal author, Dr. Robert Allen, has been involved in each of the cases — and 600 other situations wherein the normative-change process was tested and refined over a twenty-year period. You get good theory in *Beat the System*, along with the synthesized insights of long experience and disciplined retelling. In a sense, the reader is given a short course in the highly developed normative-systems program that the Human Resources Institute helps install in varied settings over a period of many months or even years.

The cases are interesting and enable the reader to appreciate how the culture-change process really works. The discussion of each step or phase is clear and persuasive, the claims realistic, and the complexities acknowledged.

There seems to be little question that the identification of existing norms and the purposeful involvement of others in the choice of desired norms, is our best hope for greater individual freedom as well as shared humanity. That being the case, *Beat the System* has to rank as *the* handbook for readers with a conscious commitment to health via wellness lifestyles.

Weaknesses

It would be helpful to have a book just like this focused exclusively on building healthy cultures in assorted medical-related institutions, as well as wellness-culture designs in schools, churches, and the workplace. These are barely mentioned in *Beat the System* (the term wellness is used once in the text), though the applications seem clear enough. But then, this was not the intended focus of the current work, and the topic will no doubt be explored in a future opus, given the recently developed health-promotion program organized by Dr. Allen and the Human Resources Institute entitled "Lifegain."

Put *Beat the System* on your "must read" list.

Allen, Robert F. *Lifegain.* New York: Appleton-Century-Crofts, 1981.

Lifegain is an organized, tested system for creating environments conducive to a wellness lifestyle. It helps you examine culture traps, the effects of adverse influences upon everyday behaviors, and strategies for gaining freedom from the tyranny of worseness norms.

There are seven steps to the *Lifegain* program. In nine chapters, Allen applies these *Lifegain* steps to describe getting fit, dealing with smoking, eating wisely, staying slim, using alcohol moderately (if at all), avoiding accidents, learning relaxation, achieving effective relationships, and getting the most from health resources. The seven *Lifegain* steps are understanding your cultures (specifically negative health influences), getting the facts, building supportive environments, putting a plan into action, keeping track of progress, rewarding yourself and having fun, and reaching out to others.

Every chapter contains a variety of questionnaires to test your awareness of the facts about each subject addressed (e.g., fitness, nutrition, etc.) and to help you recognize prevailing norms of the culture(s) which affect your thinking and behavior. Allen supplies a reading list for further study and an outline for applying *Lifegain* to your organization or community.

Strengths

There is nothing else like *Lifegain* in the wellness literature. The system is just a framework, not a blueprint, but that is precisely what most managers need to establish workable health promotion programs. The value of *Lifegain* if the theory and practical application of normative or value change to make wellness lifestyles logical, not heroic, choices. Allen describes in articulate and persuasive fashion the impact of cultures which we take for granted, and shows the way to achieve group support for *sustaining* rather than just initiating good intentions.

Lifegain is far and away the best reading available on the wellness dimension of environmental sensitivity.

Weaknesses

Lifegain is the name of a business, a trademark for Dr. Allen's program for implementing the wellness concept. For readers of the book, the ideas, principles, and opinions are the elements of value. Unfortunately, *Lifegain* as a term is sometimes employed to the point where the book seems like an extended advertisement for the business.

A lesser complaint is that Dr. Allen's celebrated wit emerges less than expected in a somewhat dry discussion of the program. A notable exception can be found in the chapter on how to get along with yourself and others. In a checklist of signs that tell if you need professional help, Allen asks fourteen questions, including: "Are you performing activities that are weird?" No guides to weirdness are provided, but presumably those who are will know.

Of all the books recommended, this is near the top of the list.

Brilliant, Ashleigh. *I May Not Be Totally Perfect, But Parts of Me Are Excellent.* Santa Barbara, CA: Woodbridge, 1979.

Why is Ashleigh Brilliant's book on the wellness honor roll of recommended publications? Let me count the ways: (1) it is a terrific collection of philosophical cartoons; (2) most of the cartoons apply quite nicely to issues of worseness and wellness (as the introduction to Day Six, on self-responsibility, indicates); (3) a well-developed sense of humor is an important aspect of mental and emotional well-being; and (4) Brilliant's "Potshots" will activate your sense of humor.

Brilliant is always wry and witty — and occasionally he is profound. His book contains just a sampling of his total production of cartoons, which at press time contained about 1,400 cards. It is organized into twelve topical sections, each introduced by the author with (expected) whimsy and self-deprecation. He also provides an interesting self-portrait entitled "How Do I Do?"

A few sample "Potshots" are in themselves the best way to represent the flavor of Brilliant's work, although the effect is much greater when accompanied by the author's clever illustrations:

- One possible reason why things aren't going according to plan is that there never was a plan.
- To be sure of hitting the target, shoot first and, whatever you hit, call it the target.
- I want all my posthumous medals in advance.
- Sometimes the best medicine is to stop taking something.
- Confidentially, I have nothing worth hiding.
- I'm ready to give up the struggle, but can't find anybody to surrender to.

Strengths

The collection of "Potshots" by subject category and the rare opportunity to read "Brilliant sentences" of greater length than seventeen words (the author's self-imposed limit) are two special qualities of this artist's work. Contrary to the low esteem which some social observers hold for the general public, Brilliant believes the maligned masses will give "total attention to any subject, no matter how profound, so long as you present it with wit, intelligence, and compassion, and discuss it fully from all sides in no more than seventeen words."

I especially enjoyed reading about Brilliant's beginnings, early career, and current personal reflections on each of the selected Potshot themes.

Weaknesses

No complaints. A fine selection for your wellness herbal-tea or carrot-juice table.

In case you wondered, the author states in the first section of his book that "Ashleigh Brilliant is my real name." What's more, he holds a genuine Ph.D. (History, University of California at Berkeley, 1964).

Dyer, Wayne W. *Your Erroneous Zones.* New York: Avon, 1976.

A guidebook to self-actualization, Dyer's book is in the tradition of Harry Browne's *How I Found Freedom In An Unfree World* (which is my all-time favorite of the genre). Follow Dyer's advice in *Your Erroneous Zones* and you will focus on attitudes and behaviors that promote happiness and personal effectiveness while minimizing the emotional red tape that parents, friends, and the culture have unwittingly wrapped around you.

Dyer's book attempts a great deal. He believes (as I do) that change is possible and that you can choose to develop and enjoy: (1) a mind of your own; (2) an openness to new experiences; (3) control over feelings; (4) the power of self- or inner direction; (5) freedom from justice and fairness traps; (6) elimination of hero worship and dependency relationships; (7) an openness to the unknown; (8) doing without blame, fault, shoulds, guilt, and worry; (9) the ability to fail successfully; and (10) a capacity to set up conditions for growth instead of chasing after the repair of deficiencies (which is the single greatest problem with the U.S. health-care system). As you can see, this is an ambitious book. Dyer describes how you can become the architect for your own best potentials as well as the doctor for healing bad habits. The first step is to design and cast a supportive environment within yourself.

Dyer's special message is that you hang on to behaviors that do not serve you because, at some level, there is a "payoff" for doing so. Usually, the payoffs are security and safety through adherence to a comfortable, learned response (however self-destructive), which relieves you from having to take charge and responsibility for what is happening. Two themes run throughout the book which apply to your efforts to shape a wellness lifestyle: (1) you are the sum total of your choices (e.g., responsibility for what you are and how you feel is yours); and (2) you must take charge of your present moments (it is the only moment in which you can experience anything — don't waste time on past and future events and expectations).

Strengths

There are so many useful lessons — this book is truly a gem. It is so good for purposes of shaping the mental and emotional images of a wellness lifestyle that I paid my teenaged daughter to read it! We would read one chapter at a time, make notes, and discuss the ideas for as long as required to understand each other's perspective on the issues involved. It was a good experience and a sound investment in my child's well-being. We got to practice the integration of Dyer's theories into the context of our own lives and, in the process, learned more about each other. I have also used sections of the book with groups of young people. No doubt about it — the topics are of vital interest.

· Dyer has a warm conversational prose style and a talent for organizing the material in a way that not only evokes agreement and understanding, but also helps you prepare to act upon new insights. The format in each chapter is a presentation of the substantive material, examples of ineffective behavior, a complete listing of payoffs for staying with self-defeating patterns, and strategies or specific recommendations and rehearsals for adopting and implementing new thought and behavior patterns. The best exercises are those designed to build positive self-images, confidence, independence, forthrightness, courage, and good feelings.

· High on the ranking of strengths are Dyer's arguments regarding the uselessness of blame, guilt, worry, being "right," and the expectation of justice in an unfair world. There are payoffs in everything you do, including being unhappy, down, or otherwise locked in worseness. Dyer helps you to consciously look at the returns on the above patterns compared with wellness alternatives. In doing so, Dyer shows that worseness choices are not very attractive. The case is persuasive that you can control your thoughts and thus your feelings and thereby the extent of your happiness and ability to pursue a wellness-oriented existence.

· The suggestion to eliminate the words "hope," "wish," and "maybe" are also well-taken. These words are procrastination devices or symptoms of "putting-it-off" habits. Change sentences like "I hope to start exercising on a regular basis" to "starting right now, I will make fitness a part of my life."

· I appreciate Dyer's distinction between not succeeding in a particular endeavor and failure as a person. The author argues that failure does not exist — it is simply someone else's opinion of how an act should be completed. You do not have to "do your best" in every single act in life (what's wrong with a mediocre bike ride?). The main point is an important one: never confuse so-called temporary setbacks with self-worth.

· Other strengths are the author's emphasis on the value of a sense of humor, his definition of intelligence as living an effective and happy life in the present moment of every day, and his definition of love as an ability and willingness to allow those you care for to choose for themselves.

· Finally, a positive comment should be made about the clever manner in which Dyer has summarized all the lessons of erroneous zone avoidance in a concluding portrait of a person who lives outside of such worseness zones. It is another glimpse at what a wellness lifestyle can look like — much like Maslow's discussions of the self-actualized person.

Weaknesses

· The only major problem I found was that Dyer does not encourage readers to look at erroneous-zone traps in three wellness dimensions — nutrition, fitness, and stress management. At times, he comes close — such as in the description of the person who has eliminated the erroneous zones (they are not sickly . . . don't believe in colds . . . treat their bodies well). I would have appreciated more on a wellness lifestyle, especially in the strategy sections of each chapter.

· A minor complaint — why did Dyer consent (or conspire) to the placement of such a ridiculous photo of himself on both the front and back covers of the book? Is he smiling or growling — hiding a bald dome or flaunting it? One side or the other would be tolerable — but both sides is too much.

A superb book. Read it and realize that you can make choices for wellness and away from erroneous "worseness" zones — right now — if you *choose* to do so.

Shanor, Karen. *The Shanor Study: The Sexual Sensitivity of the American Male.* New York: The Dial Press, 1978.

This is the first X-rated book to make the wellness honor roll. It is a report based on over 4,000 questionnaires and interviews designed and administered by the author to a cross section of American males. The interviewees' responses and Shanor's interpretations are never dull or clinical; it is doubtful that quotations will be printed in your family newspaper — which, of course, is a reflection on the sorry state of censorship, inhibition, guilt, and denial that permeates the entire area of human sexuality. *The Shanor Study* is intended as a profile of contemporary male preferences, experiences, and attitudes; the author's intent is to help us see ourselves as whole persons. Shanor believes that the data suggests we all have a great potential for love and sensuality; by better understanding and accepting our sexuality we can expand our capacity for guilt-free giving and taking in our relationships with ourselves and others.

The material is organized into all the areas or issues surrounding human sexuality you would want to know about — and maybe a few you would rather not. These include, but are not limited to, orgasm, masturbation, the varieties of male fantasies, antidotes to middle-aged boredom (massage parlors, mate swapping, prostitution), oral and anal sex, infidelity and bondage. Chapters are also devoted to sexual characteristics of certain age categories (teens, twenties, thirties, forties, and "golden years"), personal questions (e.g., your first sexual experience, position preferences), and the author's views on what lies ahead regarding the quality of relationships between males and females.

Strengths

The highest value of this book from a wellness perspective is the recognition it gives the reader that he or she is not alone, perverse, or uniquely incompetent in sexual matters — and that it is OK to evolve at your own pace in your own time. The culture, the norms, and the quality of information that we get on sex leaves a lot to be desired. We can all gain, especially when attitudes and habits are developing, from understanding that our innate and higher preferences involving tenderness, feelings, intimacy, genuineness, and other characteristics of humanistic relating are even more satisfying than the games we otherwise have to play for ourselves and others.

Another strength of *The Shanor Study* is that it is compelling as well as insightful reading. Some of the responses may seem delightfully prurient, others will be surprising (e.g., I did not know that *men* were faking orgasms), and still other excerpts could dismay even the sexually liberated.

You cannot read this book without appreciating the fact that our sexual preferences, techniques, and expectations vary enormously, while our fundamental adjustment problems and human needs are shared widely. Who has not at some time felt guilty about sex fantasies, wondered about his adequacy in satisfying a partner, or otherwise experienced fears and doubts?

Some of the author's opinions will be of particular interest, such as her statement that most "to-sleep-with or not-to-sleep-with" decisions are made in the first ten minutes of any male/female first meeting. Another thought-provoking section deals with the similarities and differences between the sexes. Perhaps the strongest part of the book is the author's summary entitled "Coming Together." In this concluding section, Shanor interjects her own interpretations from the data, and outlines a philosophy for the reader who would be a constructive, affectionate, and sensually awakened individual capable of more rewarding personal choices.

Weaknesses

The Shanor Study will freak some readers, though these are often the people who could most benefit from a tolerant reading of other sexual ways and norms. The most serious problem is the author's claim that a variety of wonderful transformations are occurring in the sexual and other relationships between males and females (e.g., more sincerity, more concern for each other, more sensitivity). All this may be true, but Shanor's data do not support the conclusion. The excerpts may or may not be representative; you have to wonder if the men who would respond to such a personal questionnaire and/or interview are a true reflection of the American male population.

Reading this book will convince you that wellness has many interesting possibilities.

Packard, Vance. *The Hidden Persuaders.* New York: Pocket Books, 1957.

This classic still deserves a reading. It reveals the diverse ways that advertisers come at you with enticements for all manner of goods that are usually neither useful nor good for you. The favored territory of these professional, skilled pitch-persons is your unconscious. *The Hidden Persuaders* describes how Madison Avenue gets women to spend nearly half again as much as they intend to spend in supermarkets, how whiskey and cigarette hucksters appeal to our hidden needs and motives, and the discouraging implications of all of this for the average person's prospects for a healthy lifestyle. Naturally, the two best reasons to understand the games of psychology professors converted into merchandisers of low-level worseness are: (1) to more effectively see through and thus ignore or laugh at their ruses; and (2) to develop counterstrategies equally as clever to promote appropriate messages for saner, life-enhancing lifestyles.

Strengths

Packard makes the worst of the hidden persuasion techniques less effective simply by raising our awareness of what is being done, which is the ultimate strength of the book. A number of fundamental questions are raised, such as, "What is the morality of manipulative advertising strategies aimed at":

- Encouraging the housewife to be a nonrational and impulsive (junk) food shopper?
- Exploiting hidden weaknesses and frailties, such as your dread of being different, latent aggressive feelings, childhood hang-ups, and sexual desires?
- Manipulating small children to help sell products to adults?
- Fund-raising for charities by subtle appeals to our desire for raised self-esteem?
- Encouraging public attitudes toward wasteful resource-consumption patterns?

Just by raising these questions, Packard helps you to avoid being used by purveyors of useless gadgetry, worseness food, empty candidates, and other products and ideas that could be hazardous to your health.

Another quality of *The Hidden Persuaders* which you might enjoy is the description of specific ad campaigns, and the backstage type of insight gained about the way "motivational analysts" interpret our characters to those with something to sell. For example, the Marlboro cigarette people were persuaded that a tattoo would be just the thing to convey a virile, masculine, "man-sized flavor" image of their cancer-producing product. However, they did not want to lose their female addicts in the process, so the slogan became, "A man's cigarette that women like too." The experts believed that you would respond to the ads by thinking that, if you smoke Marlboros, you will have a "terrifically exciting personality." Most would laugh at such notions if the appeal were open, but the talent of the hidden persuaders is to express powerful images indirectly. Another example of how far some advertisers will go was the pitch by one TV sponsor for vitamin pills. The pitch was made by a "trusted" adult figure, one Dr. Francis Horwich, "principal" of the pre-school show called the "Ding Dong School," who discussed how pretty the red pills were and how easily they could be swallowed. Children were urged to take the pills just "like I do." Another example is a detailed look at the Republican campaign strategy in the 1956 presidential election, in which the candidates were merchandised like a breakfast cereal.

Weaknesses

The major problem with this book is that it is loaded with extremely dated references, which make it seem more historical than timely. Some readers might get the idea that these things are not done today, twenty-plus years after *The Hidden Persuaders* was written. This would be unfortunate, because the techniques are not only still in use, but have greatly improved over the intervening decades.

The Hidden Persuaders was a useful book when it first appeared. The lessons and resulting immunity from advertising trickery it promotes make it still worthwhile for present purposes.

Tager, Mark, and Jennings, Charles. *Whole Person Health Care.* Portland, Oregon: Victoria Publishers, 1978.

Whole Person Health Care is intended for everyone with an interest in holistic health, high-level wellness, or any of the major dimensions of wellness. It is especially targeted for persons with these concerns who live in the northwestern part of the U.S., where the authors reside. For the benefit of the latter, a special section is included — a directory of professionals engaged in health-related work compatible with the philosophy expressed in the book. In addition, a proliferation of specific examples based on local cases are cited to illustrate the principles and suggestions put forth.

Physician Mark Tager and self-care enthusiast Charles Jennings have "put it all together" in this publication. *Whole Person Health Care* contains vignettes on innovative holistic-health practitioners, view on principles of holistic- (or "whole-person") health care, several chapters on self-care elements and techniques, and lengthy discussions on nutrition, fitness, and stress dimensions consistent with shaping a wellness lifestyle. Of special interest are sections often overlooked in health-promotion books: chapters on sexual self-care, home care for children, health activism, a glossary on alternative health options or uncommon modalities (Tai Chi, iridology, meditation, and fifty-four others), and a special report on X-rays. As an introduction to wellness or holistic health, this is one of the best. What holds a wellness lifestyle together, what provides the "wellness glue" as the authors call it, is a positive enthusiasm for living — not any particular technique or practice.

Strengths

One way I judge a book is the extent to which I deface it. That is, when I enjoy and am impressed with what I read, I underline, circle, and/or write in the margins ideas which the authors have stimulated for me. Thus, a marked-up book signals that it meant something for me, that it had an impact. No used-book store would be interested in my copy of *Whole Person Health Care* — I defaced it badly.

For starters, you will probably appreciate the tone, style, and irreverent but benign wit that Tager and Jennings employ to express their viewpoints. They do not dwell upon the negative, but do acknowledge individual differences, and provide a thorough list of choices and options in every phase of a healthy, enjoyable lifestyle.

The "personal health hazards questionnaire" is an effective consciousness-raiser that subtly introduces the specific implications of a wellness lifestyle in everyday circumstances and events.

In addition to solid content, you get treated to quite a few entertaining expressions, such as:

- "Ten slightly 'off-the-wall' ways to wind down" (one of which is to make love . . ."so slowly that the ice melts before it hits the river").
- "Stress is too serious not to be taken lightly."
- "Are you monogamous, polygamous, or just plain loose?"
- (For those who desire a "whole person" relationship with a provider)". . . take a careful look in the hand mirror which he or she gives you."

Tager and Jennings do not shy from controversy where they believe your health (and theirs) is at risk. The sections devoted to the hazards of nuclear power and excessive use of X-rays for diagnostic purposes are hard-hitting, unconventional, and enlightening.

The "home health library" of annotated book references is well chosen — many of the selections (e.g., Carlson, Fuchs, Illich, Lappe, Williams, Leonard, Benson, et al.) are standard readings for persons interested in shaping health-promoting lifestyles.

The values reinforced make a great deal of sense, particularly: (1) the ancient maxim "do no harm" and its implications in the context of holistic health; (2) time is the great healer; (3) treat the person, not the symptom; (4) the true role of the doctor is as teacher; (5) a respect for nature; (6) less reliance on medical "breakthroughs" (i.e., magic bullets); (7) a humanistic, people orientation; (8) health care as the care we take in living our lives so that we retain our health and enhance our well-being; and (9) health itself as an art form, a life-skill acquired through study and discipline which is mastered by practice.

I especially enjoyed the distinction drawn between what passes for quality medical care as contrasted with quality whole person health care, as well as the "rules" for democratic health care; how to write your doctor a letter; ways to help your doctor be more effective for you (e.g., tell him/her what you want — symptomatic cure, pain relief, high -level wellness, or what?); and the choice between "hard" and "soft" paths of modern health care.

In the overall analysis, however, I found the chapters on nutrition and "whole-person care" for kids to be, in themselves, worth the price of admission. The nutrition chapter highlights the way kids get ripped off by the sugar hustlers and provides a comprehensive and clearly understandable overview on sugar, salt, oils, coffee, processed food, vitamins, vegetarianism, fasting, and recipes for "home cooking," thrown in for good measure. Young people should especially enjoy the chapters addressed to them — and the out-front, no judgement or BS-counsel on whole-person sex!

Weaknesses

Alas, perfection is hard to find these days (and, no doubt, in other days past and future) — and who needs it, anyway, except perfectionists. But don't be one — you will have more fun not having to live up to such unrealistic expectations. Regarding the shortcomings of *Whole Person Health Care* (some of which, of course, you may think are strong points), there are but a few quibbles.

The vignettes in the overview section concerning holistic-health practitioners who are "digging wholes in the (northwestern) health-care field" are disappointing in that most seem folksy but not especially innovative.

The "wellness bag" is in fact primarily a bag of doctor-type tools for self-care, not health enrichment.

At times, Tager and Jennings dwell excessively on symptoms of low-level worseness (diseases and high-risk behaviors).

There are occasional editing problems that distract now and then (as when a meal breaks down "much more slow" and when the authors' pal Jeffrey Bland is twice introduced as "the leading nutritional biochemist in the Northwest").

The inadequate descriptions of holistic health, wellness, and naturopathy (omitted entirely) in the "57-variety-health-option" glossary — and the curious inclusion of surgery as an option in this context (are not the other fifty-six *options to* surgery — and drugs?).

Overall, however, these lapses (if they are lapses) are almost unnoticeable in the flow of this good book. It does not feel right to end on a negative note given the high quality of this Wellness honor roll

publication. Thus, let vintage Tager-Jennings style and substance express a more upbeat conclusion in an excerpt that was, for me, the
single most important counsel in the outstanding chapter on whole
-person nutrition:

> "When evaluating the quality of our meals, we must con-
> sider also the subtle touches that give them a distinctively
> human quality: a bouquet in the center of the table, soft lighting,
> grace before dinner, special music, pleasant companionship,
> and so on. These things add no vitamins or protein to the meal,
> but they nourish us nonetheless."

Ryan, Regina Sara and Travis, John W. *Wellness Workbook.* Berkeley,
Ca.: Ten Speed Press, 1981.

Just as there is (much) more to health than the absence of illness, so,
too, is there more to breathing/communicating/eating/playing/finding
meaning/moving/transcending/thinking/sensing/and feeling than you
(or certainly most people) might have imagined. Such is the promise,
the performance, and the fascinating content of this seminal contribution to the wellness philosophy by the "Pope of Wellness," — His
Eminence The Well Doctor Travis, and co-author Regina Sara Ryan.

The *Workbook* provides yet another perspective (complimentary) on
the basic skill dimensions (nutrition, stress, and fitness.) More important, it conveys a convincing message in every chapter that nearly
everything of consequence to success as a "whole person" relates to
learning to love, to embrace responsibility, and to channel life energies
toward spiritual wellness.

Wellness is defined and described at length as a choice/decision
toward optimal health, as a way of life, as a process, and as an integration of body, mind and spirit.

The *Workbook* contains about a hundred interesting diversions from
the captivating text; these include boxed-off vignettes from each author's personal stories in the context of diverse issues (e.g., John's
journal as a medical student — presented in the midst of a discussion of
the problems of the medical system.) It is also loaded with cartoons,
models, charts, quotes, diagrams, an activity profile, and a health
hazard/risk index. To top everything off, the last page consists of a
"Grand Certificate" recognizing the reader to be a "Wonderbarus Per-
sonus." Everyone familiar with the late, nearly great Wellness Resource Center operated by Travis for seven years realizes the importance of achieving W.P. status; others will quickly catch on.

If, after 240 pages of twelve chapters, three appendices, and a few
pages of wellness product ads you have not had enough, take heart:

you are now ready for the *Wellness Workbook for Helping Professionals.* Here, Travis alone describes the personal, theoretical, and practical issues from his past, present, and futuristic perspectives. It is in this work that John hints at the kind of concerns that account for his presence today in Costa Rica in pursuit of the "Gaia Hypothesis" or eternal spirit connecting us with each other and all forms of life, as John expresses his current commitment at "merging individual and planetary wellness."

Strengths and Weaknesses

The greatest strength of Travis' work (and, for some, the source of insufficient acceptance and impact) is his trail-blazing originality. This usually takes the form of controversial "new age" thinking on issues that are quite distant from the medical, health or even holistic mainstream. To read Travis (and Ryan in the *Workbook*) is to be either dazzled and convinced, challenged and provoked, or confronted and turned off. Take your pick, discover where you are, and use what you can.

Personally, I enjoyed and benefited from the *Workbook.* I think it is as valuable to the beginner as to the wellness cognisenti, savants, heirophants, and true believers.

My two favorite parts of the *Workbook* were: (1) the asides, the personal stories, charts, and tests; and (2) the humore throughout. The highlight of the latter is surely the "Wellness Antidote," a 102 point questionnaire *counter quiz* to the "Wellness Index" which "gauges your ability to break your seriousness about wellness."

To summarize my recommendation about the *Wellness Workbook:* "Don't leave the bookstore without it."

Ardell, Donald B., and Tager, Mark. *Planning for Wellness: A Guidebook for Achieving Optimal Health.* Dubuque, IA: Kendall/Hunt Publishing Co., 1982.

It seems fitting if immodest to conclude this honor roll critique as I started it, namely, with a work of my own, in this case a different kind of book written with Mark Tager, co-author of *Whole Person Health Care,* noted above.

Planning for Wellness is, as the title suggests, a guidebook for active participation in shaping your own wellness lifestyle. It was written as a tool for use in wellness seminars to assist people in making lifestyle change a practical reality at home, work, and play.

The twin focus of the *Guidebook* is on culture change and the development of a personal wellness plan.

Strengths

Naturally, none of this is objective, nor is anything else in this (or most other) books. Still, it is true that our *intent* in writing *Planning for Wellness* was that the strengths of the opus would be that it be entertaining, practical, motivational, easy to use, and effective.

Weaknesses

None, of course! How could you think such a thing? Well, truth is it remains to be seen if that which works so well in seminars is as effective when charming Mark and gentle Don are not on the scene with encouragements and proddings, interpretations and group processes.

Here is a list of possible shortcomings of *Planning for Wellness*:
- Our "true believer" spirit overwhelms the reader
- Our style is too "flippant" — we are not "serious" enough
- We do not cover the five dimensions of wellness in sufficient detail, believing (perhaps falsely) that the details have been widely available elsewhere in recent years
- Not everybody likes to do games, exercises, processes, and other tests and self-assessments — and the *Guidebook* is loaded with them, and
- There are not enough photos of the authors in living color.

Overall, we are delighted with the way the book turned out and has been received, and have found that it is very helpful for those who are teaching or otherwise communicating wellness to others.

Parting Words

I thank you for the time and confidence you placed in *14 Days*. I hope it has measured up to your expectations and my promises.

Do try to look on wellness as a process that outweighs in value the final product — however healthy and whole and self-directed you become as the years pass. It is *just* a tool or, as suggested, a Game, for moving toward your own peaks and heights. As a process, wellness will help you sustain your initial motivation. It will channel your enthusiasm, help you set purposeful directions and stay on course while extending your choices. In short, it will enable you to find more and greater life satisfactions.

From the high spots of wellness, you can enjoy the realization of your best potentials for physical, emotional, and spiritual health. From here, you can constantly experience a zest for living while flourishing with a genuine sense of well-being. In any event, never doubt that you deserve absolutely nothing less than a position at your own apex. Go for magnificence.

Consider that one of the surest and most rewarding approaches to what has been called spiritual wellness, a deeper sense of completion and meaning, is often occasioned from entering wellness into the service of man and womankind. Further, contributions to others can be contagious. Before you know it, these good attitudes and habits could spread like a virulent contagion — and before long we would experience an epidemic of well-being. So, now that you have contracted wellness yourself, begin to surround your life in a garden or greenhouse of well-being with people, places, jobs, and things that are so oriented.

Perhaps, in the course of writing so much about my favorite subject, high-level wellness, I have been too harsh on its opposite, low-level worseness. In thinking about it a bit more, maybe I should recognize that such a miserable situation is actually no worse than, say, mussels out of season. Or, a mishap with a small nuclear device.

Best wishes, friend. May you enjoy the quest for your own unique pathways to whole-person excellence.

Be well.

Index

14 DAYS TO A WELLNESS LIFESTYLE

PERSONAL CHECKLIST

The lessons of 14 Days *are:*

- [ ] **1.** Learn the rules of the Wellness Game and how to win at health and life.

- [ ] **2.** Establish where you are on the Worseness/Wellness Continuum in order that you can chart your progress in the weeks to come.

- [ ] **3.** Recognize the "health" care system for what it is: a fine resource for illness care when used appropriately but not relevant to health in the wellness sense of the word.

- [ ] **4.** Understand the power of norms and cultures and their influence in your current behaviors and future attempts to reach your best potential.

- [ ] **5.** Develop clear pictures or images in your mind of what it means to be a healthy person in a psychological or spiritual sense.

- [ ] **6.** Begin a training program that will lead to a "black belt" status or mastery in self-responsibility.

☐ **7.** Know the adequacy requirements of and the payoffs to be derived from physical fitness.

☐ **8.** Eat for optimal performance as well as enjoyment and disease avoidance.

☐ **9.** Understand the dynamics of stress management and principles for effectiveness in channeling stress energies.

☐ **10.** Learn and practice two vital stress-management skills: deep breathing and progressive muscle relaxation.

☐ **11.** Develop visualization capabilities for relaxation, creativity, health enrichment, and personal fulfillment.

☐ **12.** Know your wellness vital signs in order to monitor your progress toward the outer reaches of optimal functioning.

☐ **13.** Entertain the possibility of performing a "heroic act" in order to escalate your participation in and satisfactions from a wellness lifestyle.

☐ **14.** Develop and begin to carry out a personal wellness plan.

RECOMMENDED MUSIC TO ACCOMPANY
YOUR 14 DAYS

Day One: Mozart, *Serenade No. 6 in D Major, "Serenata Notturna"*
Day Two: Vivaldi, *The Four Seasons*
Day Three: Tchaikovsky, *Violin Concerto in D Major*
Day Four: Giuliani, *Concerto for Guitar and Strings*
Day Five: Haydn, *Lira Concerto No. 5 in F Major*
Day Six: Mendelssohn, *Violin Concerto in E minor No. 64*
Day Seven: Beethoven, *Sonata for Piano and Violin No. 1 in D Major*
Day Eight: Telemann, *Suite in G Major*
Day Nine: Handel, *Concerto No. 1 in G minor*
Day Ten: Bach, *Double Concerto in D minor*
Day Eleven: Foubler, *Marlboro Variations*
Day Twelve: Mozart, *Serenade in G Major, "Eine kleine Nachtmusik"*
Day Thirteen: Schubert, *Quintet in A Major for Piano and Strings, "Trout"*
Day Fourteen: Bach, *Brandenburg Concertos*